EFFECTIVE HEMOSTASIS IN CARDIAC SURGERY

A Society of Cardiovascular Anesthesiologists Monograph

Edited by:

Norig Ellison, M.D.

Professor and Acting Chairman,
Department of Anesthesia,
University of Pennsylvania,
Philadelphia, Pennsylvania

David R. Jobes, M.D.

Associate Professor of Anesthesia,
University of Pennsylvania,
Philadelphia, Pennsylvania

1988

W. B. SAUNDERS COMPANY

Harcourt Brace Jovanovich, Inc.

Philadelphia, London, Toronto, Montreal, Sydney, Tokyo

W. B. SAUNDERS COMPANY
Harcourt Brace Jovanovich, Inc.

The Curtis Center
Independence Square West
Philadelphia, PA 19106

Library of Congress-in-Publication Data

Effective hemostasis in cardiac surgery.

(A Society of Cardiovascular Anesthesiologists monograph)

1. Heart—Surgery. 2. Hemostasis, Surgical. 3. Hemostatics. I. Ellison, Norig. II. Jobes, David R. III. Series. [DNLM: 1. Heart Surgery. 2. Hemostasis, Surgical. WG 169 E27]

RD598.E33 1988 617′.412 88–3157

ISBN 0–7216–2757–9

Editor: Lisette Bralow

Production Manager: Frank Polizzano

Manuscript Editor: Keryn Lane

Indexer: Dorothy Stade

Effective Hemostasis in Cardiac Surgery ISBN 0–7216–2757–9

Last digit is the print number: 9 8 7 6 5 4 3 2 1

Publication Committee of the Society of Cardiovascular Anesthesiologists

CONTRIBUTORS

V. PAUL ADDONIZIO, JR., M.D.

Associate Professor of Cardiac Surgery, University of Pennsylvania. Staff, Cardiothoracic Surgery, Hospital of the University of Pennsylvania; Staff, Thoracic Surgery, Veterans Administration Hospital, Philadelphia, Pennsylvania.

Platelet Function Alterations During Cardiac Surgery; Heparin-Induced Thrombocytopenia: Diagnosis and Management

FREDERICK W. CAMPBELL, M.D.

Assistant Professor of Anesthesia, University of Pennsylvania. Assistant Anesthesiologist, Children's Hospital of Philadelphia, and Hospital of the University of Pennsylvania, Philadelphia, Pennsylvania.

Platelet Function Alterations During Cardiac Surgery

NORIG ELLISON, M.D.

Professor and Acting Chairman, Department of Anesthesia, University of Pennsylvania.
Senior Anesthesiologist, Children's Hospital of Philadelphia, and Hospital of the University of Pennsylvania, Philadelphia, Pennsylvania.

Heparin Therapy During Cardiac Surgery; Effective Hemostasis in the Cardiac Surgical Patient: Current Status

JUDITH A. FABIAN, M.D.

Associate Professor, Department of Anesthesiology, Medical College of Virginia, Richmond, Virginia.

Fibrinolytic Therapy

GLENN P. GRAVLEE, M.D.

Associate Professor, Department of Anesthesia, Head, Cardiothoracic Anesthesia, Wake Forest University, Bowman Gray School of Medicine, Winston-Salem, North Carolina.

Blood Plasma Products

MARBRY B. HOPKINS, M.D.

Assistant Professor of Pathology, Wake Forest University, Bowman Gray School of Medicine.
Medical Director of Blood Bank, North Carolina Baptist Hospital, Winston-Salem, North Carolina.

Blood Plasma Products

JAN C. HORROW, M.D.

Associate Professor of Anesthesiology, School of Medicine, Hahnemann University, Philadelphia, Pennsylvania.

Protamine: A Necessary Evil

ANTHONY D. IVANKOVICH, M.D.

The William Gottschalk, M.D. Professor and Chairman, Department of Anesthesiology, Rush Medical College.
Senior Attending and Chairman, Department of Anesthesiology, Rush-Presbyterian-St. Luke's Medical Center, Chicago, Illinois.

Thromboelastography: A Coagulation-Monitoring Technique Applied to Cardiopulmonary Bypass

DAVID R. JOBES, M.D.

Associate Professor, Department of Anesthesia, University of Pennsylvania.
Senior Anesthesiologist, Children's Hospital of Philadelphia, and Hospital of the University of Pennsylvania, Philadelphia, Pennsylvania.

Heparin Therapy During Cardiac Surgery; Effective Hemostasis in the Cardiac Surgical Patient: Current Status

JEFFREY R. KAPPA, M.D.

Instructor, Department of Surgery, University of Pennsylvania.
Fellow, Division of Vascular Surgery, Department of Surgery, University of Pennsylvania Medical Center, Philadelphia, Pennsylvania.

Heparin-Induced Thrombocytopenia: Diagnosis and Management

CHARLES J. KOPRIVA, M.D.

Professor of Anesthesiology, Yale University School of Medicine.
Director of Cardiovascular Anesthesia, Yale-New Haven Hospital, New Haven, Connecticut.

The Activated Coagulation Time (ACT)

JAMES E. LEVESON, PH.D.

Scientific Director, Special Hematology, Baylor University Medical Center, Dallas, Texas.

Fibrinolysis: A Frequent Cause of Bleeding

ALAIN J. MARENGO-ROWE, M.D., F.R.C.P., D.C.P., F.C.A.P.
Director of Special Hematology and Blood Bank, Baylor University Medical Center, Dallas, Texas.
Fibrinolysis: A Frequent Cause of Bleeding

ABDUS SALEEM, M.D.
Professor, Department of Pathology, Baylor College of Medicine.
Head, Clinical Pathology, The Methodist Hospital, Houston, Texas.
Viscoelastic Measurement of Clot Formation: The Sonoclot

ALAN JAY SCHWARTZ, M.D., M.S. ED.
Associate Dean for Academic Affairs and Professor of Anesthesiology, School of Medicine, Hahnemann University.
Anesthesiologist, Hahnemann University Hospital and Children's Hospital of Philadelphia, Philadelphia, Pennsylvania.
Heparin Therapy During Cardiac Surgery

SALWA A. SHENAQ, M.D.
Associate Professor, Department of Anesthesiology, Baylor College of Medicine.
Associate Staff, Fondren Brown Cardiovascular Unit, The Methodist Hospital, Houston, Texas.
Viscoelastic Measurement of Clot Formation: The Sonoclot

BRUCE D. SPIESS, M.D.
Assistant Professor, Department of Anesthesia, Rush Medical College.
Associate Attending and Director of Anesthesia for Hepatic Transplantation, Rush-Presbyterian-St. Luke's Medical Center, Chicago, Illinois.
Thromboelastography: A Coagulation-Monitoring Technique Applied to Cardiopulmonary Bypass

LINDA STEHLING, M.D.
Professor of Anesthesiology, SUNY Health Science Center at Syracuse, Syracuse, New York.
Platelet Transfusion

LAURAINE M. STEWART, M.D.
Associate Professor, Department of Anesthesiology, Medical College of Virginia.
Director of Cardiovascular Anesthesia, McGuire Veterans Administration Hospital, Richmond, Virginia.
Fibrinolytic Therapy

J. ANTHONY WARE, M.D.

Assistant Professor of Medicine, Harvard Medical School.
Associate Director of Coronary Care Unit, Cardiovascular Division, Beth Israel Hospital, Boston, Massachusetts.

Desmopressin Acetate in Hemorrhagic Conditions, with Emphasis on Use after Cardiopulmonary Bypass

FOREWORD

Few areas in clinical medicine have generated as much emotional response on the part of surgeons and anesthesiologists, based on so little fact and science, as have the etiology and treatment of intraoperative bleeding disorders in cardiac surgery. Although altered hemostasis is intentional in virtually all cases, there has been a lack of undisputed information to guide clinical care. This has led to a variety of institutional, emotional, and unscientific schemes for the management of bleeding disorders. Adding to the clinician's intraoperative dilemma has been the issue of availability and use of blood products and drugs necessary to achieve hemostasis.

Individuals who are familiar with modern military practice (especially in the Vietnam era) recognize the unique yet poorly defined value of fresh warm blood when infused from donors into critically ill bleeding recipients. Attempts in the 1970's to replicate the beneficial effects of fresh warm blood led to the processing and to the zealous administration of component blood therapy. Blood components rarely live up to expectation when compared with freshly donated blood. This disappointing situation is probably due to administration of coagulation factors for which there is no need, to failure to administer components that are needed, and to the inability of processed components to function like in vivo factors.

With the advent of the 1980's, the risk of disease transmission through blood products is more apparent, if not real. Even the luxury of liberal administration of blood products in a "shotgun" approach is simply not a practice that can be currently supported. Threrefore, a better understanding of the basis of hemostatic abnormalities in cardiac surgery is essential.

Despite a continued lack of available diagnostic and therapeutic precision, this monograph reviews the current pathophysiological and iatrogenic hemostatic changes seen in cardiovascular surgery. Using this information, a nonemotional response to clinical bleeding can be formulated. There are a few points worthy of emphasis that are common to many of the chapters in the monograph. They are: (1) the common thread that platelet function abnormalities are likely to be the most frequent hemostatic defect in the cardiac surgical patient; (2) heparin, while essential at the moment, is not as benign as once thought; (3) "shotgun" therapy as currently practiced is rarely successful; (4) fibrinolysis may be more common than previously believed; and (5) perhaps most importantly, future developments in the therapy of bleeding disorders will necessitate better laboratory diagnosis with more sensitive, rapid, and reproducible test results. It is clear that prospective planning of tests and available therapy should be accomplished before the clinical need arises. It is imperative to incorporate the surgical team and blood bank and hematology personnel into prospective planning of the approach to the bleeding cardiac surgical patient.

Even though there is uniformly high quality of the invited authors' contributions to this monograph, the editors' own concluding chapter, "Effective Hemostasis in the Cardiac Surgical Patient—Current Status," stands out as a highlight.

While it is reasonable to expect better diagnostic techniques and drugs for managing the bleeding cardiac surgical patient in the future, this monograph provides a current state-of-the-art review of the clinical problem. I hope this book will occupy an important place in the library of all members of the cardiac surgical team.

D. David Glass, M.D.
Professor of Surgery (Anes.) and Medicine
Chairman, Department of Anesthesiology
Dartmouth Medical School
Hanover, New Hampshire

CONTENTS

CHAPTER
1 **HEPARIN THERAPY DURING CARDIAC SURGERY** 1
Norig Ellison, David R. Jobes, and Alan Jay Schwartz

CHAPTER
2 **PROTAMINE: A Necessary Evil** 15
Jan C. Horrow

CHAPTER
3 **FIBRINOLYSIS: A Frequent Cause of Bleeding** 41
Alain J. Marengo-Rowe and James E. Leveson

CHAPTER
4 **FIBRINOLYTIC THERAPY** 57
Judith A. Fabian and Lauraine Stewart

CHAPTER
5 **BLOOD PLASMA PRODUCTS** 69
Glenn P. Gravlee and Marbry B. Hopkins

CHAPTER
6 **PLATELET FUNCTION ALTERATIONS DURING CARDIAC SURGERY** 85
Frederick W. Campbell and V. Paul Addonizio, Jr.

CHAPTER
7 **PLATELET TRANSFUSION** 111
Linda C. Stehling

CHAPTER
8 **HEPARIN-INDUCED THROMBOCYTOPENIA: Diagnosis and Management** 123
Jeffrey R. Kappa and V. Paul Addonizio, Jr.

CHAPTER
9 **DESMOPRESSIN ACETATE IN HEMORRHAGIC CONDITIONS, WITH EMPHASIS ON USE AFTER CARDIOPULMONARY BYPASS** 137
J. Anthony Ware

CHAPTER
10 **THE ACTIVATED COAGULATION TIME (ACT)** 155
Charles J. Kopriva

CHAPTER
11 **THROMBOELASTOGRAPHY: A Coagulation-Monitoring Technique Applied to Cardiopulmonary Bypass** 163
Bruce D. Spiess and Anthony D. Ivankovich

CHAPTER
12 **VISCOELASTIC MEASUREMENT OF CLOT FORMATION: The Sonoclot** 183
Salwa A. Shenaq and Abdus Saleem

CHAPTER
13 **EFFECTIVE HEMOSTASIS IN THE CARDIAC SURGICAL PATIENT: Current Status** 195
David R. Jobes and Norig Ellison

INDEX 203

CHAPTER 1

HEPARIN THERAPY DURING CARDIAC SURGERY

NORIG ELLISON, DAVID R. JOBES, and ALAN JAY SCHWARTZ

McLean looked for a procoagulant and found heparin.[1] Chargoff and Olson attempted to develop a long-acting heparin in 1938 by adding protamine to heparin, hoping for an effect similar to the long-acting protamine-zinc-insulin combination, and thereby discovered heparin's antidote.[2] By such fortuitous accidents, anticoagulant therapy evolved to the point where we now have heparin, which is essential for safe cardiopulmonary bypass (CPB), and heparin's antidote, protamine. There are three main reasons for the long lag between the discovery of heparin and its clinical application: lack of a purified preparation, poorly understood indications for its use, and lack of an effective antidote.[3]

Heparin therapy in general medical practice has been divided into three categories according to the goals and doses: mini-, moderate, and maxidose. The last regimen is the only one applicable in cardiac surgery, where the goal is total hemostatic paralysis.[4]

HEPARIN DOSE SCHEDULES

Prior to 1975 heparin therapy was based on rigid dose schedules that varied greatly between institutions without any obvious explanation for the variation. In that year two classic articles by Bull et al. demonstrated clearly that there was a wide variation in patient response to heparin therapy both in sensitivity and in duration.[5, 6] The former signifies the degree of prolongation of a measured test of coagulation, the latter indicates the half-life. Bull et al. found that sensitivity varied 3-fold and duration varied 4-fold, indicating that there may be as much as a 12-fold

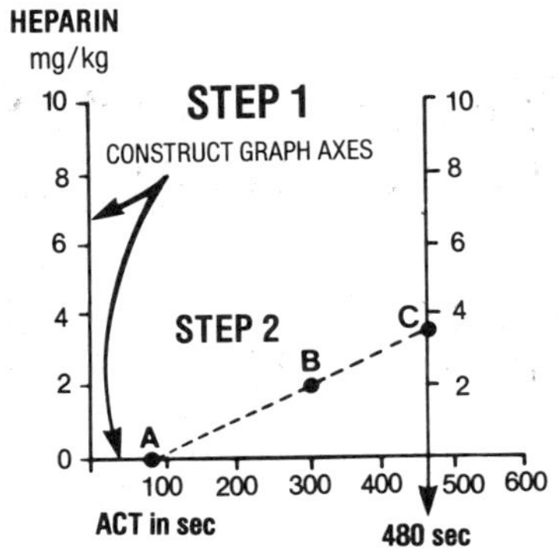

STEP 2

Determine initial ACT (A) and administer 2 mg/kg heparin.

Then, measure ACT (B) and plot both values.

Extrapolate an imaginary line through "A" and "B" to intersect with 480 sec line to find point "C."

Example:—3.5 mg/kg heparin is needed to produce 480 sec ACT, or 1.5 mg/kg in addition to the 2 mg/kg heparin already given.

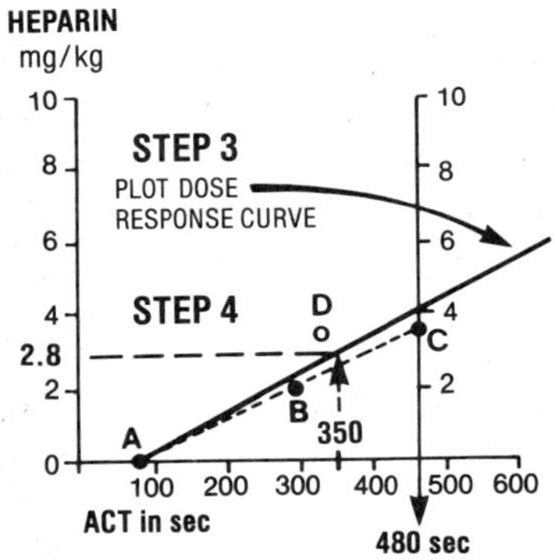

STEP 3

After required heparin has been given, measure ACT. Plot point "D."

If point "D" does not superimpose on point "C," then a dose response curve is drawn from "A" to a point midway between "C" and "D."

STEP 4

After 60 minutes, measure the ACT. Determine amount of heparin in patient's circulation from the dose response curve.

Example:—Assume an ACT of 350 sec: the heparin level would be 2.8 mg/kg. To return to 480 sec, 1.2 mg/kg of heparin is needed.

STEP 5

To reverse anticoagulation, circulating heparin level is determined as in Step 4. The neutralizing dose of protamine is heparin level mg/kg × 1.3.

Example:—ACT of 325 sec is measured. Heparin level is 2.6 mg/kg, and 3.4 mg/kg protamine is required.

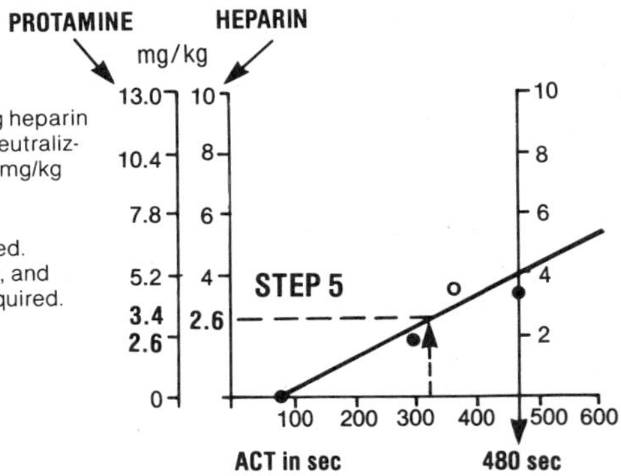

Figure 1–1. Procedure for construction and use of the dose-response curve in heparin therapy. ACT = Activated coagulation time. (From Bull BS, Huse WN, Brauer FS, Korpman RA: Heparin therapy during extracorporeal circulation. II. The use of a dose-response curve to individualize heparin and protamine dosage. J Thorac Cardiovasc Surg 69:685–689, 1975.)

variation in individual patient response to a given dose of heparin. To accommodate this individual patient variation, Bull et al. introduced the concept of heparin titration (Fig. 1–1), in which a patient's response to a subtotal dose of heparin is determined. Additional heparin is administered to be certain that the activated coagulation time (ACT) has been prolonged sufficiently. After subsequent doses are administered, the ACT is rechecked to confirm adequate anticoagulation.

One of the controversial areas in heparin therapy in cardiac surgery has been the definition of the goal before institution of bypass. Stated simply, the goal of therapy is to achieve sufficient hemostatic paralysis so that thrombogenesis will not occur during exposure to the foreign surface represented by the pump during CPB. Bull's goal was to maintain the manual ACT between 300 and 480 seconds. Below 300 seconds the risk of thrombogenesis is real; but the definition of the upper limit is less fixed. Bull et al. point out that above 600 seconds the end point is quite irreproducible and suggest that platelet-mediated hemostasis will suffer some derangement, thereby making the patient more susceptible to intracranial bleeding.

The studies conducted by Bull et al. were carried out using a manual ACT. For reasons primarily of convenience (Table 1–1), the automated ACT has largely replaced the manual test and has been used by several investigators to extend the original concept of heparin titration. In 1978 Young et al. reported that keeping the automated ACT greater than 400 seconds would prevent microscopic coagulation, using as their end point the appearance of a fibrin monomer.[7] Shortly thereafter we compared the automated ACT to our standard monitoring device, a manual protamine titration, and concluded that as long as the automated ACT was greater than 300 seconds, anticoagulation was adequate for CPB.[8]

We were unable to demonstrate a linear heparin dose–ACT response relationship as originally reported by Bull et al., particularly when the ACT was excessively prolonged (Fig. 1–2). Cohen examined this relationship in a rigorous statistical manner and demonstrated conclusively that a two-point dose-response curve remains statistically valid and clinically useful throughout cardiac surgery as long as the automated ACT is less

TABLE 1–1. CHARACTERISTICS OF THE IDEAL OPERATING ROOM TEST OF HEMOSTASIS

1. Only simple maneuvers are necessary to obtain reproducible results.
2. Minimum equipment, which is compact, inexpensive, and quiet, is required.
3. Result is available quickly, even with abnormally prolonged time.
4. Test is performed on whole blood rather than plasma.
5. Test reagents are stable indefinitely.
6. Test must not require prolonged attention away from operator's usual duties.

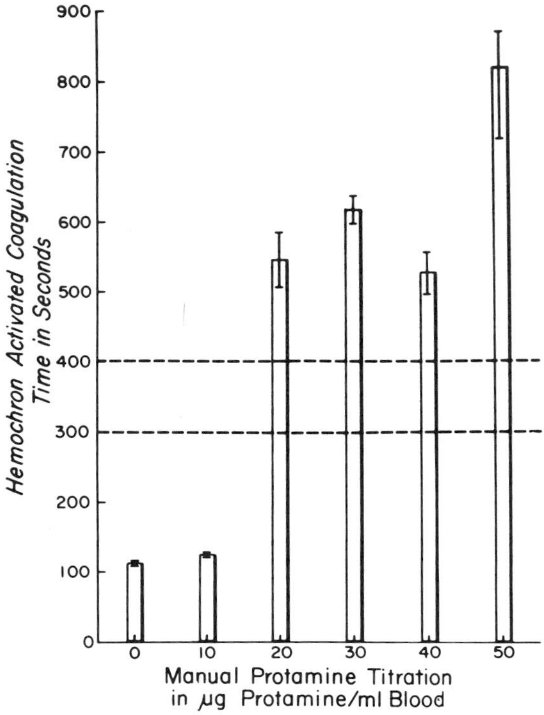

Figure 1–2. Automated activated (Hemochron activated) coagulation time versus manual protamine titration. On the horizontal axis, milliliters of blood is that amount required for optimal neutralization. Note the marked increase at 20 µg of protamine per milliliter of whole blood. (From Jobes DR, Schwartz AJ, Ellison N, et al.: Monitoring heparin anticoagulation and its neutralization. Ann Thorac Surg 31:161–166, 1981.)

than 500 seconds.[9] Beyond that value the relationship is not linear, but anticoagulation is adequate.

Mammen et al. point out that a clear difference in data becomes apparent when comparing reports concerning extensive fibrinolysis following CPB published before 1970 with more recent papers in which only slightly elevated fibrin split products were observed.[10] Borderline or inadequate anticoagulation may result in low-grade activation of coagulation and produce secondary fibrinolysis. Therefore, the observations of Mammen et al. may be explained by the introduction and widespread acceptance by the mid-1970's of the concept of heparin titration to a defined end point, thereby resulting in uniform adequate anticoagulation.[11] This same point has also been made by Bull: "The major risk is not too much heparin but too little, with the precipitation of disseminated intravascular coagulation (DIC)."[12] The major emphasis on risk of insufficient heparin must be tempered, however, to also avoid unwarranted excess. It must be remembered that the dose of heparin dictates the dose of protamine. Large doses of protamine are associated with increased postoperative bleeding.[13] Complement activation is substantial during cardiac surgery and peaks following protamine administration.[14, 15] Toxic effects of protamine are partially dose-dependent.

The appropriate dose of heparin for infants and small children has not been evaluated as comprehensively but follows the same principles as for adults. The initial dose response has not been well-documented in infants and children. The use of profound hypothermia and the reduced capability of infants to metabolize and excrete heparin prolong the effects of initial heparin doses. Monitoring of heparin effect can significantly reduce the amounts used compared to fixed protocols. We employ the same ACT of 400 seconds as an indication of adequate heparin therapy in children.

TESTS OF HEPARIN THERAPY

Heparin therapy inhibits the action of four activated coagulation factors: IIa (thrombin), IXa, Xa, and XIa (Fig. 1–3). In the usual clinical doses for other than cardiac surgery, the goal is to prolong the activated partial thromboplastin time (aPTT) to 2 to 2½ times normal. Since Factor IXa is the most sensitive to heparin therapy and its action is inhibited by smaller doses than the other three activated factors, the aPTT—a test of the intrinsic system—is the logical test to measure the effect of heparin in moderate doses. However, with the dosage used in CPB, the aPTT is prolonged infinitely. Nevertheless, after protamine reversal of heparin, the aPTT would be a logical, sensitive test to detect the presence of any small residual quantity of heparin. The failure of the aPTT to gain widespread acceptance in this area is most certainly a reflection of the fact that the aPTT is an inconvenient test for use in the operating room.

The Lee-White whole blood coagulation time (WBCT) was originally described in 1903 by two men, one of whom (Paul Dudley White) went on to receive greater recognition in cardiology than in hematology.[16] This was the first test used to measure the effect of heparin therapy. However, except for requiring minimal equipment and being inexpensive, this test failed to meet most of the characteristics required of the ideal intraoperative test of hemostasis (Table 1–1). The WBCT was abandoned for two reasons. First, the test required prolonged attention away from the anesthesiologist's usual duties. Second, the results were obtained too late. For example, a WBCT of 30 minutes would indicate 30 minutes after sampling that additional heparin was required 30 minutes earlier. Two modifications restored the WBCT to surgical use: automated measurement and shortened time to end point. Schriever et al. demonstrated that the relationship between the WBCT and the automated ACT could be expressed by the following formula:[17]

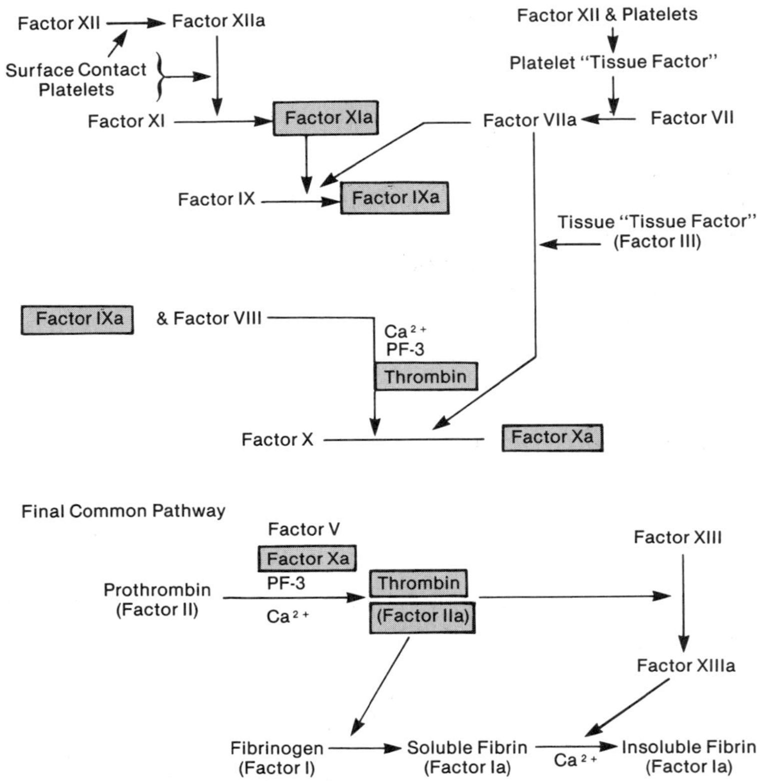

Figure 1–3. Coagulation cascade and its interrelationships. The four activated factors that are inhibited by heparin—IIa (thrombin), IXa, Xa, and XIa—are enclosed in boxes. This cascade demonstrates the interrelationships between extrinsic and intrinsic pathways in the first stage of coagulation. (The concept of separate pathways is no longer valid.) PF-3 = Platelet factor 3. (Adapted from Ellison N, Jobes DR, Schwartz AJ: Implications of anticoagulant therapy. Int Anesthesiol Clin 20:121–135, 1982.)

$$\text{WBCT (min)} = (\text{ACT in secs}/2.5) - 45$$

In this equation, a WBCT of 30 minutes would be equal to an automated ACT of 187 seconds. Thus, in the example above, the same information obtained in 30 minutes would now be provided in 3 minutes. The automated ACT, which is a relatively gross test, fulfills the characteristics listed in Table 1–1 and, in addition, has stood the test of time.

Hattersley introduced the ACT of whole blood in 1966 as ". . . a simple, reliable and reasonably sensitive bedside test of the coagulation mechanism" and stated that "immediate activation of freshly drawn blood by an inert diatomite greatly shortens the coagulation time (normal mean, 1 minute 47 seconds; standard deviation, 13 seconds) and produces a rather sensitive test for coagulation defects."[18] Although the ACT was a giant step forward from the Lee-White WBCT, today the ACT is considered a poor screening test of the intrinsic system and informative only if significantly prolonged—e.g., factor levels greater than 1.0 per cent of normal will usually provide normal values.[19] As reported by Hattersley, Factor VII levels and platelet deficiencies are not detected by the ACT. Because of these intrinsic limitations, the ACT has been replaced in large measure by the aPTT as a screening test. Why then has the ACT attained such great popularity for monitoring anticoagulation with heparin during CPB? The introduction of automated ACT devices, in which electrical, magnetic, mechanical, or optical means are used to detect the end point, has resulted in a very convenient method of monitoring the effect of administrated heparin on the coagulation mechanism. For the anesthesiologist who is concerned with the administration of anesthesia and other drugs, with ensuring adequacy of ventilation and normovolemic status, and with monitoring hemodynamic values, the convenience of the automated ACT is probably paramount in explaining its widespread acceptance.[20]

Prolongation of either the aPTT or the ACT is not specific for heparin, a fact that must be remembered when trying to control bleeding following CPB. To confirm the presence of heparin, either a protamine titration or a direct heparin assay must be used. In the former the ability of small doses of protamine (e.g., 10 μg/ml of blood) to shorten a prolongation of the measured test is used to confirm that the prolongation is due to heparin; in the latter a colorometric assay is used. Until recently heparin levels were determined indirectly by the response to protamine titration. The ability to measure plasma heparin concentrations directly by means of the activated Factor Xa assay permitted Esposito et al. to confirm the work of earlier investigators who used less sophisticated indirect methods (Fig. 1–4).[21] While direct assays have contributed to a better understanding of the pharmacokinetics of heparin, most clinical testing is directed at assessing the in vivo anticoagulant effect because that is the effect that will determine if thrombus formation during CPB has been successfully inhibited. Logically, this determination is best accomplished by the actual inhibition of clot formation.[4]

The question of heparin-specific effect can readily be answered by means of a protamine titration, which can be performed in a qualitative or quantitative manner. In the qualitative test, 10 μg of protamine is added to one of two test tubes, to each of which 1.0 ml of blood is subsequently added. If blood in the tube containing protamine clots first, heparin was present and was neutralized so that the blood clotted. Conversely, if the blood in the tube containing no protamine clots first, heparin was not present and the protamine exerted an in vitro anticoagulant effect on the blood in the other tube. By adding protamine to

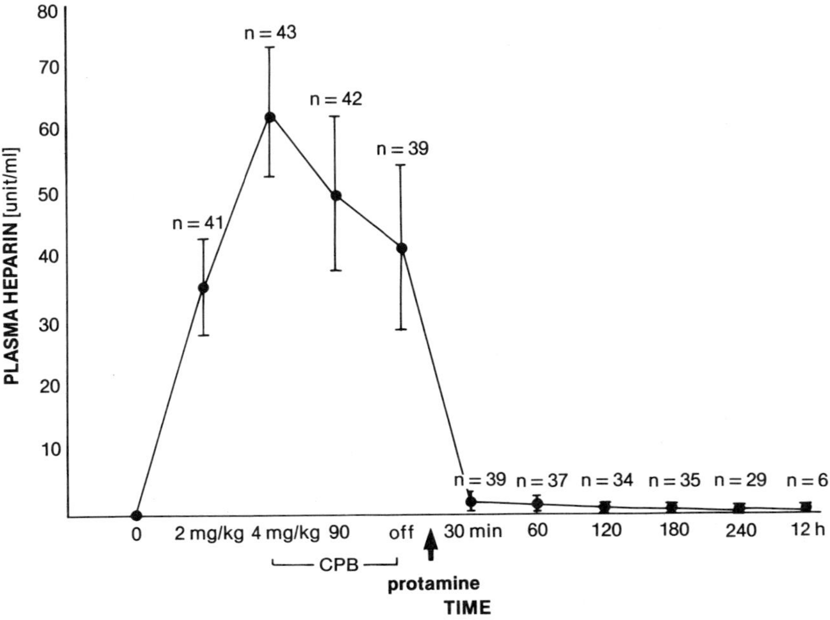

Figure 1–4. Plasma heparin levels throughout cardiopulmonary bypass (CPB) and following heparin reversal. Each point represents the mean plasma heparin concentration ± standard deviation as determined by an automated synthetic substrate assay. (From Esposito RA, Culliford AT, Colvin SB, et al.: The role of the activated clotting time in heparin administration and neutralization for cardiopulmonary bypass. J Thorac Cardiovasc Surg 85:174–185, 1983.)

several test tubes in 10 μg increments, usually from 0 to 50 μg, this test can be made quantitative. Multiplying the concentration in the test tube in which the blood clots first by the patient's estimated blood volume will determine an accurate protamine dose to be administered to neutralize the heparin effect. If the tube containing no protamine clots first, there is no heparin effect and protamine administration is not indicated.

The disparity between heparin dose, concentration, and clinical effect appears to be multifactorial in origin, with weight, volume of distribution, preoperative anticoagulation status, age, hemodilution, and hypothermia all potentially modifying the dose relationship.[18] Variation in heparin lots and other unidentified patient variables undoubtedly also contribute. The observed disparity argues strongly not only for individual titration of heparin and protamine therapy but also for verifying that the desired ACT response has been achieved after heparin administration and before commencement of CPB. Similar confirmation is required after protamine administration and before chest closure.[11]

HEPARIN RESISTANCE

Heparin resistance is the term used to describe the state in those patients in whom the administration of conventional heparin doses (300 units/kg) produces a negligible effect on coagulation. The usual gaussian distribution of heparin dose–ACT responses will result in some patients demonstrating a mild insensitivity that merely represents the lower end of the clinical response to heparin (Fig. 1–5). However, some patients will demonstrate a lack of response that is well below the 95 per cent confidence limit.[22] Marked heparin resistance in a given patient can be due to several different etiologies acting separately or in combination, and frequently no etiology is obvious (Table 1–2). Anderson recently reported a patient with multiple etiologies (heparin pretreatment, low antithrombin-III [AT-III] level, intraventricular thrombus, coronary artery disease) who required 1700 units/kg to achieve adequate anticoagulation for CPB.[23]

Sabbagh et al., without attempting to identify the etiology of heparin resistance in their patients, treated them with fresh frozen plasma (FFP)

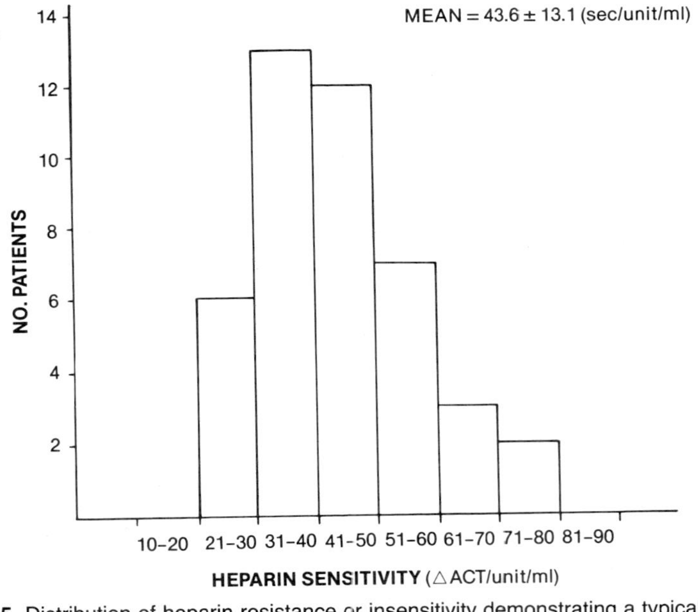

Figure 1–5. Distribution of heparin resistance or insensitivity demonstrating a typical gaussian distribution. (From Esposito RA, Culliford AT, Colvin SB, et al.: The role of the activated clotting time in heparin administration and neutralization for cardiopulmonary bypass. J Thorac Cardiovasc Surg 85:174–185, 1983.)

TABLE 1–2. ETIOLOGY OF MARKED HEPARIN RESISTANCE

1. Ongoing active coagulation.[11]
2. AT-III deficiency, congenital or secondary.
3. Previous heparin therapy.[22]
4. Drug interaction as with oral contraceptives.
5. Presence of other medical syndromes such as hypereosinophilia or coronary artery disease.[11]
6. Drug error in dose, route of administration, or product. (Not a true cause of resistance, but must always be considered.)[8]
7. Advanced age.[31]

References for specific entries are noted.

and successfully decreased heparin requirements to the normal range.[24] While acknowledging that their solution was an empirical one, they pointed out that FFP is the only source of AT-III and has been used in patients with hereditary AT-III deficiencies to decrease heparin requirements. AT-III is a plasma protein that binds with heparin, resulting in a marked acceleration of the process whereby thrombin and other serum proteases are inactivated.

The consequence of not recognizing and correcting heparin resistance prior to the onset of CPB is unlikely to be catastrophic thrombosis. Low-grade activation of coagulation leading to consumption of platelets and procoagulants is more likely to occur. This can result in microemboli whose effect will vary depending upon where they lodge, or in a hemorrhagic diathesis following the termination of CPB because of platelet and procoagulant consumption. The possible occurrence of either catastrophic thrombosis or low-grade coagulation activation is further argument for abandonment of fixed heparin protocols and for ensuring that a safe level of anticoagulation has been demonstrated before commencing and during maintenance of CPB.

HEPARIN IN UNITS VS. MILLIGRAMS

Unlike most drugs, heparin is neither chemically nor biologically homogenous. The common denominator of the chemically related sulfated mucopolysaccharides called heparin, which vary in primary sugar sequence, molecular weight, and charge, is that they share a measurable net "anticoagulant" activity defined by very specific in vitro assays.[25]

Heparin exhibits a potency between 90 and 110 per cent of USP Heparin Units and is prepared, assayed, and dispensed only in terms of units per milliliter.[26] The continued description of heparin doses in milligrams is not only incorrect but dangerous, for it may lead to under- or overdosing a patient by a factor of 10. The prevalence of this error in the terminology is perhaps best exemplified by the fact that several of the references in this review describe their heparin dose in terms of milligrams. Much confusion concerning heparin dose would be eliminated if heparin doses were always correctly described in terms of units.

HEPARIN ADMINISTRATION

Heparin, in contrast to its antidote protamine, has minimal cardiovascular effects. For this reason, heparin can safely be administered rapidly as a bolus via a centrally located line. Aspiration of blood before and after heparin administration will confirm that the heparin has been administered into the vascular system. This practice may be safely substituted for direct injection into the right atrium by the surgeon.

HEPARIN REBOUND

The term "heparin rebound" was originally used to describe a state of hypercoagulability that follows the discontinuation of heparin therapy. The opposite inference is made in the context of cardiac surgery. In 1956 Kolff et al. first described heparin rebound as "a treacherous phenomenon in which heparin is neutralized by protamine sulfate and the clotting

TABLE 1–3. CHRONOLOGY OF THEORETICAL EXPLANATIONS FOR HEPARIN REBOUND

Year	Explanation
1957	Heparin may be released by red blood cell breakdown.
1958	Heparin may escape from the circulation into the extravascular space and return via the lymphatics and thoracic duct to the circulation many hours later, after protamine has been administered and cleared.
1959	Heparin may be injected into tissues instead of intravenously, forming a depot source for prolonged absorption.
1961	A part of the heparin level may be temporarily neutralized by an endogenous antagonist, not otherwise specified. When this antagonist is cleared from the blood, heparin activity is then demonstrated.
1962	Protamine may be metabolized or combined with other plasma proteins before heparin is removed.
1966	Protamine chloride does not produce heparin rebound, although protamine sulfate does. This may be due in part to the more rapid metabolism of protamine sulfate.
1970	Heparin rebound is seen more commonly with hypothermia. It had previously been shown that heparin levels do not decay as rapidly during hypothermic perfusions.
1974	For a given heparin level, low levels of platelets result in a more pronounced effect of that heparin level on the coagulation mechanism. Since thrombocytopenia is a common occurrence following open heart surgery, it is quite possible that heparin activity may be enhanced.
1981	Careful monitoring post-cardiopulmonary bypass with an automated protamine titration will detect heparin rebound more frequently.

Adapted from Ellison N, Beatty CP, Blake DR, et al.: Heparin rebound, studies in patients and volunteers. J Thorac Cardiovasc Surg 67:723–729, 1974.

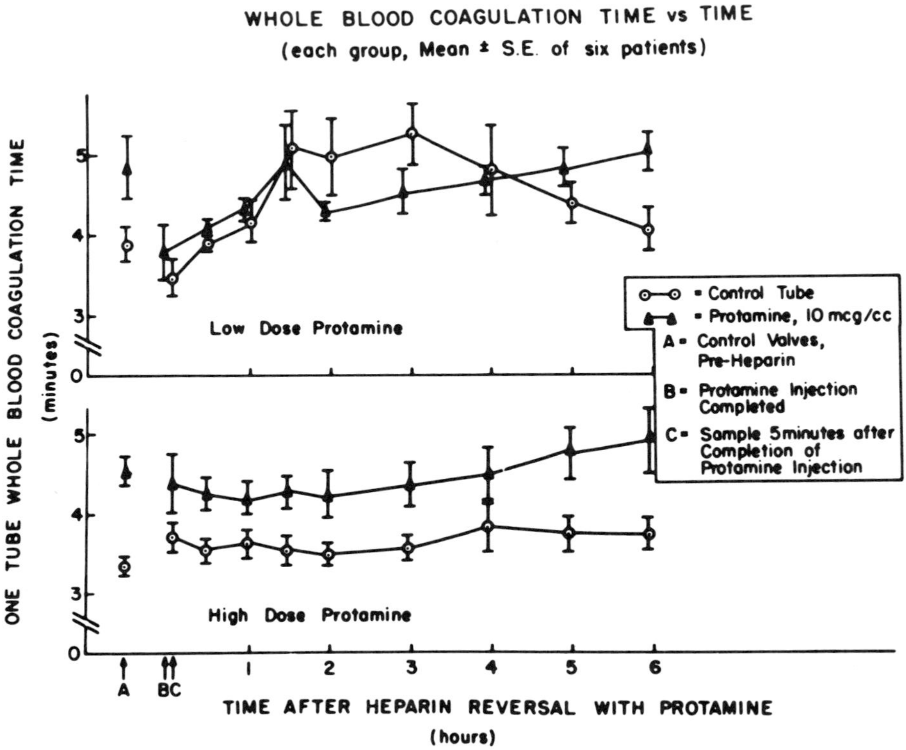

Figure 1–6. Whole blood coagulation time versus time following heparin neutralization for two groups of patients following open-heart surgery. For the low-dose protamine group, the average whole blood coagulation time for the tube with protamine added was shorter than that for the control tube (between 1½ and 4 hours)—demonstrating that heparin rebound had occurred. At no time was this reversal in the whole blood coagulation time seen in the high-dose protamine group. Results are statistically significant ($p < 0.05$) in the low-dose protamine group only for the control tubes (point A) and for the measurement at 6 hours; in the high-dose protamine group, all determinations were significant except immediate reversal (point C) and measurements at 1 and 4 hours. (From Ellison N, Beatty CP, Blake DR, et al.: Heparin rebound, studies in patients and volunteers. J Thorac Cardiovasc Surg 67:723–729, 1974.)

time becomes normal in a matter of minutes. However, protamine seems to be eliminated from the blood before heparin is, thus leaving the heparin uncovered as demonstrated by protamine titration."[27] The incidence of heparin rebound has been variously reported from 0 to 50 per cent.[28, 29] The pharmacodynamics of an acutely administered drug undergoing redistribution—protamine—compared with a completely distributed drug—heparin—appears sufficient to explain the phenomenon of heparin rebound. Various other theories to explain heparin rebound are listed in Table 1–3.

Figure 1–6 demonstrates in a carefully controlled situation the occurrence of heparin rebound as demonstrated by the protamine titration in six out of six patients who received a very low dose of protamine, equivalent to 57 per cent of the heparin dose, compared with a high-dose protamine group in which 113 per cent of the heparin dose was administered. We do not believe that heparin rebound is a common occurrence. However, it is such an easily and specifically treated entity that failure to consider and look for it in a patient who is bleeding after initial heparin neutralization either in the operating room or the intensive care unit may subject patients to needlessly prolonged closures or even unnecessary re-exploration.[30]

SUMMARY

The fortuitous discovery of heparin by McLean has been followed by more than seven decades of numerous animal and human studies as well as by a wealth of clinical experience. The use of heparin is essential to prevent thrombus formation during CPB. Heparin neutralization following CPB is equally essential to permit clot formation and promote wound healing. There are four essential steps that will ensure the adequacy of heparin therapy in patients undergoing open-heart surgery:

1. Careful administration of the appropriate dose to the circulation before the institution of bypass.
2. Confirmation that coagulation is adequately prolonged before the institution of CPB.
3. Serial confirmation of adequate anticoagulation during CPB. We do this at 30-minute intervals.
4. Neutralization of heparin with protamine, and confirmation that the ACT has returned to near baseline value and/or that no circulating heparin can be detected.

References

1. McLean J: The thromboplastic action of cephalin. Am J Physiol 41:250–252, 1916.
2. Chargoff F, Olson KB: Studies on the chemistry of blood coagulation. VI. Studies on the action of heparin and other anticoagulants. The influence of protamine on the anticoagulant effect in vivo. J Biol Chem 122:153–167, 1937–1938.
3. Ellison N, Ominsky AJ: Clinical considerations for the anesthesiologist whose patient is on anticoagulant therapy. Anesthesiology 39:328–336, 1973.
4. Ellison N, Jobes DR, Schwartz AJ: Implications of anticoagulant therapy. Int Anesthesiol Clin 20:121–135, 1982.
5. Bull BS, Korpman RA, Huse WN, Briggs BD: Heparin therapy during extracorporeal circulation. I. Problems inherent in existing heparin protocols. J Thorac Cardiovasc Surg 69:674–684, 1975.
6. Bull BS, Huse WN, Brauer FS, Korpman RA: Heparin therapy during extracorporeal

circulation. II. The use of a dose-response curve to individualize heparin and protamine dosage. J Thorac Cardiovasc Surg 69:685–689, 1975.
7. Young JA, Kisker CT, Doty DB: Adequate anticoagulation during cardiopulmonary bypass determined by activated clotting time and the appearance of fibrin monomer. Ann Thorac Surg 26:231–240, 1978.
8. Jobes DR, Schwartz AJ, Ellison N, et al.: Monitoring heparin anticoagulation and its neutralization. Ann Thorac Surg 31:161–166, 1981.
9. Cohen JA: Activated coagulation time method for control of heparin is reliable during cardiopulmonary bypass. Anesthesiology 60:121–124, 1984.
10. Mammen EF, Koets AB, Washington DC, et al.: Hemostasis changes during cardiopulmonary bypass. Semin Thromb Hemost 11:281–292, 1985.
11. Ellison N: Heparin-protamine monitoring and cardiovascular effects. *In* Estafanous G (ed): Anesthesia and the Heart Patient. Stoneham, MA, Butterworth (in press).
12. Bull BS: Heparin anticoagulation (letter). Ann Thorac Surg 29:204, 1980.
13. Guffin AV, Dunbar RW, Kaplan JA, et al.: Successful use of a reduced dose of protamine after cardiopulmonary bypass. Anesth Analg 55:110–113, 1976.
14. Loubser PG: Complement activation during surgery with and without cardiopulmonary bypass (abstract). Anesth Analg 65:S–90, 1986.
15. Cavaroschi NC, Pluth JR, Schaff HV, et al.: Complement activation during cardiopulmonary bypass. Comparison of bubble and membrane oxygenators. J Thorac Cardiovasc Surg 91:252–258, 1986.
16. Lee RI, White PD: A clinical study of the coagulation time of blood. Am J Med Sci 145:495–503, 1913.
17. Schriever HG, Epstein SE, Mintz MD: Statistical correlation and heparin sensitivity of activated partial thromboplastin time, whole blood coagulation time and an automated coagulation time. Am J Clin Pathol 60:323–329, 1973.
18. Hattersley PG: Activated coagulation time of whole blood. JAMA 196:436–440, 1966.
19. Weintrobe MW, Lee CR, Boggs DR, et al. (eds): Clinical Hematology (ed 8). Philadelphia, Lea & Febiger, 1981, p 1057.
20. Ellison N: Postoperative prolongation of activated clotting time. *In* Reves JG, Hall KD: Common Problems in Cardiac Anesthesia. Chicago, Yearbook Medical Publishers, 1987, pp 449–454.
21. Esposito RA, Culliford AT, Colvin SB, et al.: The role of the activated clotting time in heparin administration and neutralization for cardiopulmonary bypass. J Thorac Cardiovasc Surg 85:174–185, 1983.
22. Esposito RA, Culliford AT, Colvin SB, et al: Heparin resistance during cardiopulmonary bypass, the role of heparin pretreatment. J Thorac Cardiovasc Surg 85:346–353, 1983.
23. Anderson EF: Heparin resistance prior to cardiopulmonary bypass. Anesthesiology 64:504–507, 1986.
24. Sabbagh AH, Chung GKT, Shuttleworth P, et al.: Fresh frozen plasma: A solution to heparin resistance during cardiopulmonary bypass. Ann Thorac Surg 37:466–468, 1984.
25. Cines DB: Heparin: Do we understand its anti-thrombotic action? Chest 89:420–426, 1986.
26. The United States Pharmacopeia, 21st revision. United States Pharmacopeia Convention, Rockville, MD, 1985, p 482.
27. Kolff WJ, Effler DB, Groves LK, et al: Disposable membrane oxygenator (Heart-Lung Machine) and its use in experimental surgery. Cleve Clin Q 23:69–75, 1956.
28. Ellison N, Beatty CP, Blake DR, et al.: Heparin rebound, studies in patients and volunteers. J Thorac Cardiovasc Surg 67:723–729, 1974.
29. Pifarré R, Babka R, Sullivan HJ, et al.: Management of postoperative heparin rebound following cardiopulmonary bypass. J Thorac Cardiovasc Surg 81:378–381, 1981.
30. Jobes DR, Schwartz AJ, Ellison N: Heparin rebound (letter). J Thorac Cardiovasc Surg 82:940–941, 1981.
31. Gravlee JP, Brauer SD, Roy RC, et al.: Predicting the pharmacodynamics of heparin: A clinical evaluation. J Cardiothoracic Anesth 1:379–387, 1987.
32. Ellison N: Heparin: New information on an old drug. J Cardiothoracic Anesth 1:377–378, 1987.

CHAPTER 2

PROTAMINE: A Necessary Evil

JAN C. HORROW

HISTORY

The steps leading from protamine's discovery to its clinical applications form an excellent example of how knowledge of molecular structure, coupled with a bit of luck, can lead to a great clinical advance. One hundred and twenty years ago, Miescher discovered protamine in the course of his investigations of the cell nucleus (a subject of great interest then as now). He identified a nitrogenous base that was bound via a salt-like linkage to the acidic nuclear material of Rhine salmon sperm[1] but failed to recognize it as a protein. Years later, Kossel isolated protamines from many other species. Together protamines formed a heterogeneous group of compounds. Following Kossel's recommendation, each protamine was named after the species of fish from which it was isolated—salmine from salmon, scombrine from mackerel, and clupeine from herring. In 1896, Kossel separated arginine and other amino acids from the protamine of Baltic sea sturgeon testes, thus establishing protamines as alkaline protein molecules.[1]

Further advances in protamine structure awaited the analytical chemistry spawned from World War I. Ando and colleagues[1] devised general methods for determining the primary amino acid sequences of protamines. Salmine, the protamine extracted from salmon gonads, was found to contain nearly 67 per cent arginine. These positively charged amino acid residues make protamine polycationic and explain the salt-like linkage with anionic phosphoric acid residues of DNA that Meischer had described in a gross fashion in 1870. Today, commercial preparation of protamine from salmon milt is achieved via a crude extraction and filtration process utilizing alcohol and sodium chloride. The drug is marketed either as a dried powder (DuPont Critical Care, Wilmington, DE) or as a 1 per cent solution (various suppliers).

Protamine is used to neutralize the anticoagulant effects of heparin and to delay the absorption of subcutaneously administered insulin. How did these clinical applications come about? Hagedorn, working in Copenhagen in the 1930's, sought a means to delay absorption of insulin following subcutaneous injection.[2] After finding that insulin–nucleic acid complexes display an acid-shifted isoelectric zone, he reasoned that the isoelectric zone of insulin might be alkaline-shifted by combining it with an alkaline molecule such as protamine. In the resultant mixture, insulin would exist as an acid and be sparingly soluble; thus, its absorption might be delayed. Hagedorn thus created the long-lasting insulin complex protamine-zinc insulin, which was later modified[3] to form isophane insulin, a pH-neutral combination of protamine and insulin also known as NPH (neutral protamine Hagedorn) insulin.

News of Hagedorn's success prompted several groups to test the ability of protamine to delay absorption of other compounds, heparin among them. Best's group in Toronto immediately began tests of the new long-acting insulin in depancreatized dogs; Jaques worked on heparin chemistry in an adjacent room. One evening, Jaques and a colleague, McCutcheon, mixed protamine with heparin. Jaques recounts that a "precipitate that looked like a plastic" appeared.[4]

Nothing came of their observation, nor of subsequent attempts by Best's group to delay heparin absorption with protamine. The next year, Chargaff and Olson, in the course of their own attempts to delay heparin absorption with protamine, reported the serendipitous finding that protamine entirely neutralized heparin's anticoagulant activity in animals,[5] thus establishing the basis for its use in man as the antidote for heparin.[6] The neutralization of heparin by protamine was subsequently found to be accomplished ionically: The polyanionic sulfated heparin combines with the polycationic arginine-rich protamine to form the stable precipitate that Jaques and McCutcheon observed.

Jaques and colleagues developed the protamine titration test,[7] in which blood heparin levels are determined by combining blood with incremental amounts of protamine and observing for clot formation. In 1956, Hurt[8] applied this technique to guide protamine dosage of heparin neutralization in the post–cardiopulmonary bypass period.

Soon after the introduction of protamine insulin, reports of anaphylactoid reactions appeared. Walther[9] reported in 1939 that three guinea pigs given intracardiac protamine died of pulmonary edema. But it was Jaques who pioneered the work on protamine toxicity.[10] His studies in various species documented the adverse circulatory effects that still plague clinicians. These effects will be discussed in detail.

Today, protamine has two clinical applications: to neutralize the anticoagulant effect of heparin, and to delay absorption of subcutaneously administered insulin. While this chapter deals with the use of protamine following cardiopulmonary bypass (CPB), it would not be complete without mentioning another potential clinical use of protamine: the treatment of malignancy. It is not surprising that a compound whose biological function is to associate with DNA might affect cell division and tumor growth. There is voluminous recent literature on the role of protamine in cellular processes. Both heparin[11] and protamine[12] can inhibit angiogenesis and decrease tumor mass in the laboratory. However, clinical trials of protamine as a treatment for malignant disease have proved unsatisfactory to date.[13] With future work to better define the desired molecular characteristics, protamine derivatives may be useful in cancer therapeutics.

RESTORATION OF CLOTTING ACTIVITY

This section will focus on three distinct issues that arise in the use of protamine as a heparin-neutralizing agent: protamine as an anticoagulant itself, heparin rebound, and how to select the appropriate dose of protamine.

Protamine as an Anticoagulant Itself

Large amounts of protamine inhibit coagulation in vitro.[7, 14–16] For this reason, administration of excess protamine has been feared as a potential cause of postoperative bleeding. In vivo, however, protamine seems to be removed rapidly from the circulation.[10, 17] Ellison et al. demonstrated that excess protamine minimally increases the Lee-White whole blood coagulation time (WBCT). After 600 mg/70 kg of protamine, the clotting time of unheparinized volunteers increased from 6.7 min to 8.2 min; the partial thromboplastin time (PTT) was not affected. In addition, the Lee-White WBCT returned to baseline within 30 minutes. When studied in patients undergoing CPB, the results were similar.[18] Is there a pharmacological basis for this small effect? Possible explanations include effects on platelets and on clotting proteins. Protamine induces thrombocytopenia in dogs[10, 19] and in humans.[20] Also, thrombocytopenia accompanies pulmonary vasoconstrictive responses to protamine in humans.[21, 22] However, because these changes in platelet count are very short-lived and extreme decreases are needed to prolong clotting times,[23] decreases in platelet count are unlikely to provide the explanation sought. Regarding platelet function, aggregation in vitro is impaired by the protamine-heparin complex,[24] although protamine alone has no deleterious effects. It has not been established that platelet dysfunction from excess protamine leads to increased bleeding in patients.

On the other hand, protamine does affect thrombin.[15] In vitro, it inhibits the ability of antithrombin-III (AT-III) to inactivate thrombin. While this may at first seem to be an effect favoring coagulation rather than inhibiting it, this effect on AT-III is thought to be due to competition of protamine with AT-III for thrombin; protamine may bind to thrombin and, thus, inhibit it. Furthermore, protamine has been shown to competitively inhibit thrombin's ability to convert fibrinogen to fibrin.[15] Concentrations of only 100 μM protamine in vitro reduce thrombin activity to below 50 per cent.

Thus, protamine does inhibit coagulation in vitro and does minimally prolong measurements of the clotting system in volunteers and in patients. However, doses needed to achieve clinical anticoagulant effects are more than double those used routinely and more than three to four times the dose shown to result in return of adequate coagulation. Because of protamine's apparent rapid disappearance,[17] and because small doses of heparin do exert an important clinical effect, it seems prudent not to withhold additional doses of protamine in moderation whenever a residual heparin effect is suspected. The danger in giving additional doses of protamine for continued bleeding is that the hemostatic defect may not be residual heparin. Thus, the search for and correction of the real hemostatic defect may be delayed or forgotten.

Heparin Rebound

This term is now used in reference to the reappearance of anticoagulant activity several hours after heparin neutralization with protamine, despite complete initial neutralization. Using an in vitro protamine titration test, protamine dose may be calculated so as to neutralize exactly the amount of heparin remaining in the circulation. When protamine was administered in that fashion, heparin rebound, as measured by repeat protamine titration, occurred in all of 12 patients between one and five hours after neutralization. When larger doses of protamine were given (based on the total amount of administered heparin), Lee-White coagulation times and protamine titrations indicated no heparin rebound.[25] Since chest tube drainage was not quantitated in that study, it is unclear whether these effects on clotting times translated into clinically significant blood loss. In contrast, when Guffin et al. gave small dose ratios of protamine to patients, chest tube drainage was significantly decreased compared with that in a group receiving the standard dose ratio.[26] Most surprisingly, the group with greater bleeding had received only about 200 mg of additional protamine. Differences in the types of coagulation tests, reagents, and techniques may be responsible for the contrasting results of these studies.[27] Kaul et al. compared two schema for administering heparin.[28] In one group, heparin was given "by the clock"; in the other, it was administered only when needed according to the results of coagulation testing. Both the reappearance of anticoagulation and excessive postoperative bleeding occurred more often with the former method. Heparin rebound appears to be a real clinical entity.

The type of heparin used for anticoagulation during bypass may itself be important in achieving adequate neutralization with protamine. Heparins are complex macromolecules with multiple components and may differ in their anticoagulant properties. For example, pork mucosal heparin has a stronger anti-Xa activity than does beef lung heparin. In one study comparing heparins, protamine restored the activated coagulation time (ACT) to normal values when either the pork or beef heparin preparation was used to anticoagulate 100 patients for bypass. However, patients who had received pork mucosal heparin bled an additional 200 ml over 24 hours compared with those who had received beef lung heparin.[29] Could protamine be better at neutralizing beef lung heparin than pork mucosal heparin? In fact, protamine's neutralizing capacity has been shown to vary among the different heparin preparations and components.[30] Protamine neutralizes the anti-IIa actions of heparin more easily than the anti-Xa actions[30]; thus, pork mucosal heparin, with stronger anti-Xa activity, may be more poorly suited as an anticoagulant when protamine neutralization will be needed, as during cardiopulmonary bypass.

Appropriate Protamine Dose for Neutralization of Anticoagulation

Nearly 15 years ago, Ellison et al. wrote that the clinically used dose ratio varies from 0 to 4 mg of protamine for each 100 units of heparin administered to the patient during bypass surgery.[18] These diverse doses remain in use today, although most centers use a dose ratio between 1 and 1.3 mg per 100 units; dose calculation is based on the total dose of heparin administered rather than on that remaining in the patient at the time of protamine administration.[31] Owing to heparin metabolism, the amount of heparin remaining in the patient at the time of neutralization is less than the total amount administered prior to and during bypass. Thus, despite the fact that hypothermia decreases heparin degradation dramatically, a protamine-heparin dose ratio of as little as 0.3 mg per 100 units can restore routine coagulation parameters to normal.[18, 27, 32]

One might ask if the best dose of protamine is the minimal amount needed to neutralize heparin. It seems clear that the important issue is not how best to pick the initial protamine dose, but rather that the adequacy of neutralization be monitored and additional drug be provided when needed. The various methods for evaluating the extent of anticoagulation and the return of adequate coagulation are discussed in another chapter. One should note, however, that the ACT is affected by dilution[29] and by hypothermia[29]; dose-response curves[33] utilizing data obtained during hypothermia may be misleading. Because clot formation using the ACT depends on platelet phospholipid, very low platelet counts also prolong the ACT.[23] Furthermore, because heparin rebound is possible, it may be optimal to administer protamine at two times following extracorporeal circulation: once after bypass, and again one or two hours later to prevent heparin rebound. The results of routine use of a second protamine dose have not been reported.

IDIOSYNCRATIC REACTIONS

Undesirable hemodynamic responses to the rapid injection of protamine were recognized soon after its introduction into clinical medicine. Within a minute or two of rapid protamine injection, systemic blood pressure decreases precipitously, as do cardiac filling pressures.[34] Cardiac output is usually maintained[35, 36] or increased[34] in patients with good ventricular function. If filling pressures are maintained by rapid volume administration, then the fall in blood pressure may be averted.[37] Within five minutes of its occurrence, the reaction is over and hemodynamics have returned to normal. This type I (Table 2–1) or hypotensive response, while undesirable, is not idiosyncratic. Since it can be elicited in most patients, it is classified more accurately as a side effect, much as nausea is a side effect of morphine. Histamine is the presumed mediator. Protamine is one of several alkaline molecules that has been shown,[38, 39] like *d*-tubocurarine, morphine, and some antibiotics such as clindamycin and vancomycin,[40] to displace histamine, which is also alkaline, from mast cells. Convincing evidence is still lacking[41] to prove that the hemodynamic effects of rapid injection of these compounds are in fact due to histamine and not to some other known (e.g., leukotriene) or as yet unknown mediator released along with histamine.

Hypotension following protamine administration has attracted great attention. A great deal of animal research, mostly in dogs, demonstrates that protamine decreases systemic blood pressure[10, 42–45] and systemic vascular resistance,[19, 46, 47] and increases pulmonary arterial pressure[19, 42, 48] and pulmonary vascular resistance.[19, 48–50] Cardiac output also decreases, mostly owing to decreased preload, since there is probably

TABLE 2–1. CLASSIFICATION OF PROTAMINE REACTIONS

Type I.	Systemic hypotension from rapid injection—a predictable response.
Type II.	Anaphylactic or anaphylactoid reaction—an idiosyncratic response.
Type III.	Catastrophic pulmonary vasoconstriction—an idiosyncratic response.

no effect of protamine on inotropy.[51, 52] These cardiovascular changes occur in conjunction with transient decreases in platelet and leukocyte counts.[19, 43] For further details of these animal investigations, the reader is referred to a recent review.[53] It is noteworthy that the pulmonary vascular changes seen in dogs do not occur routinely in humans.[34–46, 54, 55] However, pulmonary vasoconstriction can occur as an idiosyncratic response (see below).

It is only within the last decade that reports have appeared of more serious clinical sequelae, such as protracted hypotension,[56] pulmonary edema,[57] and catastrophic pulmonary vasoconstriction.[58] These reactions are listed in Table 2–2 and are discussed in order.

Diabetic Patients

Theoretically, patients may be sensitized to protamine during subcutaneous administration of protamine-containing insulins, such as protamine zinc insulin (PZI) or neutral protamine Hagedorn insulin (NPH). Not all long-acting insulin preparations contain protamine.[3] Protamine was suspected (and ruled out) as the cause of cutaneous reactions to PZI or NPH insulin long ago.[59] Moorthy et al.[56] linked use of protamine-containing insulin to cardiovascular collapse occurring after intravenous administration of protamine. They postulated that true (i.e., IgE-mediated) allergy was responsible for the reaction. Confirmation of a true allergic etiology is exceedingly difficult after a reaction has occurred. As with other reports of anaphylactic reactions, the one of Moorthy et al. also lacked confirmation. The response to their report was a plethora of case reports claiming anaphylaxis to protamine as the cause of idiosyncratic cardiovascular compromise.[60–68] In some cases skin tests were performed and were negative[60, 65, 66]; in 7 patients, skin tests were positive.[61, 65, 68] An allergic etiology is highly suspected in one of these cases[61]—a young woman developed flushing, headache, and tachycardia when rechallenged with 1 mg of intravenous protamine. In none of these cases were IgE protamine-specific antibodies demonstrated.

The data implicating allergy to protamine in diabetics are unconvincing. For example, a substantial percentage of those diabetics studied have circulating antiprotamine IgE (53 per cent)[69] or antiprotamine IgG (91 per

TABLE 2–2. CATASTROPHIC REACTIONS TO PROTAMINE

1. Reactions in patients with diabetes mellitus taking protamine insulin preparations.
2. Reactions in patients with prior exposure to intravenous protamine.
3. Reactions in patients with cross-reacting antigens.
4. Noncardiac pulmonary edema (usually delayed) after protamine administration.
5. Catastrophic pulmonary vasoconstriction.

cent).[70] One would expect a high incidence of protamine reactions in such patients. However, only one of 25 NPH insulin–dependent diabetic patients followed prospectively by Levy[71] sustained a protamine reaction, and it was of the pulmonary vasoconstrictive type (type III). Do the many case reports of protamine reactions in diabetics merely represent a bias of ascertainment? True allergy to protamine may be caused by protamine-containing insulins; good prospective data to determine just how often this might occur are still lacking.

Prior Exposure to Intravenous Protamine

Previous administration of intravenous protamine may have occurred during vascular surgery—any procedure utilizing extracorporeal circulation, cardiac catheterization, renal hemodialysis, or blood component donation (pheresis). Progress in anesthetic and postoperative medical care now permits cardiac surgery and extracorporeal circulation in patients of old age or those with advanced cardiovascular disease. As a result, it is fairly common for a patient presenting for cardiac surgery to have had previous vascular surgery, previous cardiac surgery, or even to be dialysis-dependent.

Is every patient with prior exposure to protamine at increased risk for an adverse response? Thousands of patients receive protamine during cardiac catheterization and undergo subsequent CPB. Yet, as seen in Table 2–3, there are only six case reports of patients with prior exposure to protamine and subsequent immediate idiosyncratic protamine reactions. Furthermore, a convincingly positive skin test occurred in only one of the six patients (the "positive" responses to 1:1000 protamine reported by Doolan[68] can occur in unsensitized control patients).[72] Thus,

TABLE 2–3. REPORTS OF PROTAMINE REACTIONS IN PATIENTS WITH PRIOR INTRAVENOUS PROTAMINE EXPOSURE

Author	Initial Exposure(s)	Second Exposure	Interval	Skin Tests	Comments
Best et al.	Cath•2, CABG	Cath	2 weeks	Not done	Complement-mediated
Doolan et al.	Cath•2, CABG	Cath	1.5 years	+ 1:1000	Cardiac arrest
Doolan et al.	CEA	CEA	6 weeks	+ 1:1000	Cardiac arrest; bronchospasm
Andersen	Dialysis	Dialysis	Various	Not done	BP high/low
Lakin et al.	Pheresis	Pheresis	Unknown	+ 1 ng/ml	IgG; complement-mediated
Jackson	CEA	AortoFem	2 months	Not done	Cardiac massage

Cath = Cardiac catheterization; CABG = coronary artery bypass surgery; CEA = carotid endarterectomy surgery; AortoFem = aortofemoral bypass surgery; BP = blood pressure; + = positive cutaneous response.

the role of prior sensitization in the cardiovascular collapse of five of these patients is questionable. There are prospective data relevant to this issue; Levy found only one protamine reaction in over 1500 nondiabetic patients undergoing cardiopulmonary bypass, most of whom are presumed to have received protamine during catheterization.[71]

The rarity of adverse protamine reaction during surgery (prior exposure having occurred during catheterization) may be due to an interval between exposures that does not favor protamine antibody formation. Antibody formation is unlikely to occur within a week of initial exposure, and many patients have surgery within a few days of catheterization. Allergy is more likely to occur with multiple drug exposures and with an exposure interval of about two weeks.[73] Of reported protamine reactions, the interval between drug exposures ranges from 2 weeks to 1.5 years (Table 2–3).

Patients with Cross-Reacting Antigens

Two groups of patients are at risk for protamine reactions due to potential sensitization by cross-reacting substances: patients with fish allergy, and patients with prior vasectomy. Adverse responses to protamine were reported in three patients found to be allergic to fish.[74, 75] One patient suffered syncope when eating several species of true fish,[74] and was found to have IgE antibodies to codfish determined by RAST (radioallergosorbent testing). Four pheresis donors (of 140) sustained protamine reactions; two had allergies to fish. It is not known whether these two patients had antibodies against fish protamine or against contaminating antigenic determinants.[75] Should protamine be withheld in patients with a reasonable history of allergy to true fish? Probably not—six such patients followed prospectively[76] received protamine without suffering cardiopulmonary changes.

Vasectomized men may be at risk for protamine allergy. While sperm are immunologically foreign, they are protected from attack by the immune system by a "blood-testes" barrier. Systemic absorption of sperm occurs with vasectomy, thus stimulating antibody production. Sperm-agglutinating antibodies are common (73 per cent) in vasectomized men,[77] as are autoantibodies to human protamines (22 per cent).[78] Since human and salmon protamines are quite similar,[79] the stage is set for a cross-reacting antigen—salmon protamine—to combine with human protamine antibodies. It is curious that there is only one case report of a protamine reaction.[80] This patient experienced hives and pruritus following protamine given at a cardiac catheterization performed 15 years after elective vasectomy. As with most vasectomized men, further testing revealed evidence of sperm-agglutinating antibodies and of antibodies to human protamine. This man was rechallenged with protamine months later during cardiac surgery. He was pretreated with antihistamines and corticosteroids; no reaction occurred. While this patient may well have had antibodies against fish protamine, the evidence presented is not conclusive.

Noncardiac Pulmonary Edema

A syndrome consisting of decreased pulmonary compliance and capillary leak leading to pulmonary edema with or without anasarca has been associated with CPB (and thus with protamine administration) in 20 patients.[57, 64, 81–87] Systemic hypotension, bronchoconstriction, and low left atrial pressure may accompany the reaction. The most peculiar feature of these reports is the late occurrence of this syndrome; at least 15 minutes and often one to three hours elapse between protamine administration and detection of disturbed homeostasis. Owing to this poor temporal correlation, numerous alternative explanations for this phenomenon have been suggested,[82] and rightly so! These include transfusion-related events (see Ch. 5), complement activation by extracorporeal circuits, and mediators present in albumin or plasma protein fraction. In fact, protamine is not necessary for noncardiac pulmonary edema after bypass to occur; Iglesias and Nuñez reported a case that occurred prior to the administration of protamine.[85] Protamine may be a convenient scapegoat.

Catastrophic Pulmonary Vasoconstriction

Classic protamine reactions involve systemic hypotension and massive loss of intravascular fluid to tissues via capillary leak.[53] In 1983, Lowenstein reported a subset of patients who experienced catastrophic pulmonary hypertension immediately following protamine administration.[58] Unlike the victims of anaphylactoid reactions who have low right- and left-sided filling pressures, patients with catastrophic pulmonary vasoconstriction (CPVC) had several-fold increases in pulmonary artery pressure leading to right ventricular failure and its consequences: elevated central venous pressure, low flow across the pulmonary circuit, and low left atrial pressure.

Unlike its effects in laboratory animals, protamine does not routinely change pulmonary artery pressure in humans,[36, 55, 88] nor does it affect right ventricular function.[89] As an accompanying phenomenon, platelet count decreases transiently at the start of a CPVC reaction. Normally, platelet count drops mildly (28 per cent) in patients given protamine.[20] In dogs, the thrombocytopenia is more pronounced (90 per cent decrease).[10] In one patient with mitral valve disease who sustained a CPVC reaction to protamine (Fig. 2–1), the platelet count dropped from 76,000/

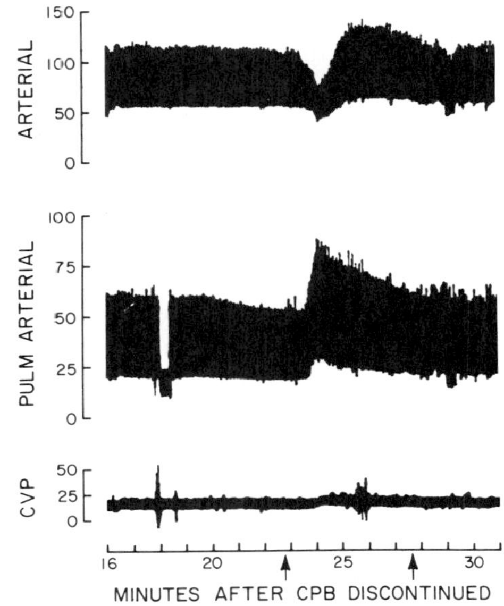

Figure 2–1. Systemic arterial, pulmonary arterial, and central venous (CVP) pressures, measured in mm Hg, in a patient who sustained a CPVC response to protamine. The left arrow on the horizontal axis indicates bolus administration of 10 mg of protamine sulfate. The right arrow indicates rechallenge with an additional 10 mg of protamine. Note that the rechallenge was benign. (From Horrow JC: Thrombocytopenia accompanying a reaction to protamine sulphate. Can Anaesth Soc J 32:49–52, 1985.)

mm^3 to $12{,}000/mm^3$ four minutes after protamine administration.[21] These features suggest[53] that CPVC following protamine is an event distinct from the anaphylactoid reactions previously described, and that the transient fall in platelet count was related either causally or as a common consequence of an as yet undescribed mechanism.[21] These expectations have been verified in an investigation of four patients who sustained protamine reactions.[22] Three of the patients sustained systemic hypotension, pulmonary hypertension, and elevated levels of the complement fragment C5a and of thromboxane, without experiencing changes in plasma histamine concentration. The fourth patient had systemic hypotension without alteration in pulmonary pressure. While C5a and thromboxane levels were unchanged in that patient, the plasma histamine level was elevated. It appears that the first three patients suffered a type III reaction, while a type II reaction was responsible for the fourth patient's difficulties. As with Horrow's patient, transient thrombocytopenia was found; more interestingly, there was transient leukopenia with a transpulmonary gradient, indicating pulmonary sequestration of leukocytes.[21] This is of interest because leukocytes play a role in complement-mediated processes and may be central to the development of adult respiratory distress syndrome.[90]

Based on this work and on work in sheep,[91] one can postulate a mechanism for type III protamine reactions. Activation of complement by the protamine-heparin complex initiates the reaction. Anaphylotoxins generated by the complement cascade result in aggregation, stasis, and pulmonary sequestration of leukocytes. Release of oxygen-free radicals, lipid peroxidation, and generation of arachidonic acid metabolites then produce thromboxane, which is responsible for pulmonary vasoconstriction.

The incidence of CPVC following protamine is not known. Morel et al. discovered it in two patients in their prospective series of 48, a rate of 4 per cent. In a less well-controlled series, Levy reported the syndrome in four patients of 1743, or 0.2 per cent.[92] The incidence of CPVC will probably vary from one practice to another. It depends on the characteristics of the patient population, since patients with baseline alterations in pulmonary hemodynamics seem to be more susceptible. It also depends on the method of protamine administration; slow, dilute infusion appears less likely to cause a catastrophic change in pulmonary pressures compared with bolus or rapid administration of the drug.

ARTERIAL VS. VENOUS INJECTION

Adverse cardiovascular responses to protamine in laboratory animals are associated with passage of the drug through the pulmonary vasculature.[42] Initial passage through the lungs can be avoided by injecting the drug into the left side of the circulation. Is left-sided injection advantageous in patients? Median sternotomy permits ready access to left atrial, left ventricular, or ascending aortic sites. However, left-sided injection of drugs cannot be endorsed without reservation; major organ dysfunction, including stroke, might occur from embolization of air, particles, or platelet aggregates[37] into the systemic circulation. Direct left-sided injection of protamine circumvents the protection provided by either the pulmonary vasculature or the bypass pump bubble traps and filters. Yet, the risk of embolism may be worthwhile if left-sided injection offers protection from adverse reactions to protamine.

Trubov et al. first reported left-sided injection in 1978,[93] followed by reports from Aris[94] and Iida.[95] Although the results of left-sided injection were favorable, none of these studies compared their results with those of a right-sided injection control group, and it is known that right-sided injection is usually benign.[54] Rogers et al.[96] demonstrated that responses in pigs to left- and right-sided injections were equivalent. This stands in contrast to a study in dogs by Wakefield et al., in which systemic hypotension occurred more often with rapid (10 sec) venous injection than with rapid aortic arch injection.[97]

In humans, Frater and colleagues[35] documented decreased systemic blood pressure and systemic vascular resistance and increased cardiac index with right-sided injection compared with left atrial administration. The right-sided group also had elevations in blood histamine concentrations. However, the histamine assay used was crude. These researchers speculated that the cardiovascular changes were related to histamine released by the lungs in response to protamine injection. But when Alaoui tried left-sided injection, two patients experienced profound systemic hypotension (40 mm Hg).[98] Apparently, Frater's group infused fluid rapidly during protamine administration to counter decreases in preload.[99]

Other studies[37, 93] have confirmed that volume infusion prevents hypotension following left-sided protamine injection. For example, Pauca et al.[37] maintained filling pressure by volume infusion when rapidly administering intra-aortic protamine to 79 patients. Cardiac output increased, while systemic blood pressure was essentially unchanged. They caution that it is essential to keep the arterial cannula in place to provide rapid volume replacement. This technique carries the additional risk of clot formation around the cannula.[37] Cherry and co-workers[100] administered protamine slowly (1 $mg \cdot kg^{-1} \cdot min^{-1}$) via either the intra-aortic or the intravenous route to 100 patients. In each group decreases in pulmonary arterial and pulmonary capillary wedge pressures accompanied a drop in cardiac index. Only the intra-aortic group experienced a decrease in systemic blood pressure, and that decrease was slight (6 per cent). These investigators found no advantage to arterial injection.

Casthely et al.[101] gave four-minute injections of protamine to dogs at 1 $mg \cdot kg^{-1} \cdot min^{-1}$ by one of three routes: left atrium, peripheral vein, or central vein. Only the central vein group experienced hemodynamic changes: systemic blood pressure and systemic vascular resistance decreased, cardiac index increased, and pulmonary arterial pressure and pulmonary vascular resistance increased. Plasma histamine concentrations increased over four-fold in the central vein group, but these increases in the other groups were not statistically significant. Since left atrial or peripheral venous infusion permits drug dilution prior to passage through the lungs, it appears that the site of injection is irrelevant as long as the drug is given slowly in dilute form.

In perhaps the most carefully controlled study of injection route using awake and anesthetized dogs, Taylor et al.[52] showed that 60-second injections of protamine into the descending aorta in awake dogs produced decreases in cardiac index, systemic vascular resistance index, systemic blood pressure, CVP, and LVEDP despite no change or small increases in contractility. Contractility was measured using end-systolic pressure-volume relationships, a new technique which, unlike dP/dt and its derived indices, is independent of changes in preload and afterload.[102]

The investigators concluded that protamine's cardiovascular effect is to decrease preload, regardless of injection site.

Left-sided injection may ameliorate the deleterious cardiovascular effects of rapid (within 2 min) protamine injection. However, the clinical scenario requiring such rapid protamine administration needs to be assessed. Left-sided injection has not been shown to be superior to slower (3 min or more) right-sided injection in preventing a type I reaction. The increased risks associated with left-sided injection, coupled with the absence of any clearly demonstrable benefit, argues for routine right-sided injections.

Does left-sided injection confer added protection from allergic (type II) or pulmonary vasoconstrictive (type III) reactions? Theoretically, type III reactions might be lessened by avoiding initial pulmonary passage. There are no data in humans, and such data will be difficult to gather owing to the sporadic occurrence of these events. The rarity of these reactions must be weighed against the possibility of embolism and stroke when choosing a left-sided injection technique.

PRETREATMENT APPROACHES

Prophylaxis

The clinician is sometimes faced with the need to administer protamine to a patient who either is in a group at questionably higher risk for protamine reaction (NPH insulin- or PZI-dependent diabetics, those with fish allergies, or men with prior vasectomy) or has a history of protamine sensitivity. One approach to management of this patient is to administer protamine but to provide prophylaxis to counter its adverse effects. Owing to the heterogeneity of adverse responses with multiple suspect mediators (histamine, thromboxane, and unknown others), one should identify the specific concern and tailor prophylaxis accordingly. Watson et al. were faced with the need to give protamine to a patient undergoing cardiac surgery who had a high likelihood of producing antibodies to human protamine owing to prior vasectomy.[80] The patient received steroids and diphenhydramine immediately prior to protamine injection and suffered no adverse sequelae. Of course, this does not prove that the patient would have had a protamine reaction without prophylaxis, nor does it prove that prophylaxis prevented a reaction.

One might postulate that prostaglandin synthetase inhibitors might protect against thromboxane-mediated CPVC reactions. In dogs given acetylsalicylic acid, thrombocytopenia was not ameliorated; however, the elevated pulmonary arterial pressure and pulmonary vascular resistance were blunted.[19]

The hazard of relying on prophylaxis is seen in a report from Brauer.[103] He gave cimetidine, diphenhydramine, and hydrocortisone prior to the induction of anesthesia to a man who had suffered an anaphylactoid reaction to protamine during cardiac catheterization. After CPB, a three-minute intra-aortic protamine injection resulted in pulmonary hypertension, systemic hypotension, and the need for cardiac massage. Here, a probable type III reaction occurred when prophylaxis was directed against a type II reaction. There are two lessons from this report. First, the mediators of the various protamine reaction types are probably different; prophylaxis needs to be tailored to the type of reaction suspected. Second, one cannot assume that systemic hypotension is histamine-mediated and can thus be averted with antihistamines.

A similar approach by Campbell[104] was more successful. His patient had experienced hypotension, urticaria, and facial numbness following a protamine injection during cardiac catheterization. The patient received prednisone, cimetidine, and diphenhydramine, once prior to an attempted percutaneous transluminal angioplasty and then again during the following emergency coronary bypass procedure. No adverse reaction occurred following protamine administration to that patient.

A Priming Technique

Wakefield and colleagues postulated that a pretreatment dose of protamine might ameliorate its adverse effects. In their investigations in dogs,[97, 105] 0.75 $mg{\cdot}kg^{-1}$ protamine was administered rapidly three minutes prior to 150 $units{\cdot}kg^{-1}$ of beef lung heparin. A second group of dogs received saline pretreatment instead of protamine; and a third group received 3 pretreatment doses of protamine (each 0.75 $mg{\cdot}kg^{-1}$) given 7, 5, and 3 minutes prior to heparin, respectively. All dogs in the third group required additional heparin to achieve a thrombin time over 100 seconds. All the animals received a neutralizing dose of 1.5 $mg{\cdot}kg^{-1}$ protamine 30 minutes after heparin.

The pretreatment scheme appeared to ameliorate the cardiovascular effects of reversal doses of protamine in these animals. Systemic blood pressure decreased sharply in the saline group, only mildly in the 0.75 $mg{\cdot}kg^{-1}$ pretreatment group, and very little in the thrice-pretreated group. Heart rate decreased and pulmonary artery pressure increased only in the saline group. An apparent biphasic drop in systemic blood pressure (Fig. 2–2) in the saline group prompted the investigators to speculate on multiple mechanisms of the response to protamine: a first phase involving direct vasodilation and drop in systemic vascular resistance, and a second phase wherein platelet aggregation engenders release of vasoactive substances responsible for subsequent pulmonary hypertension, bradycardia, and additional systemic hypotension. In support of this theory, the

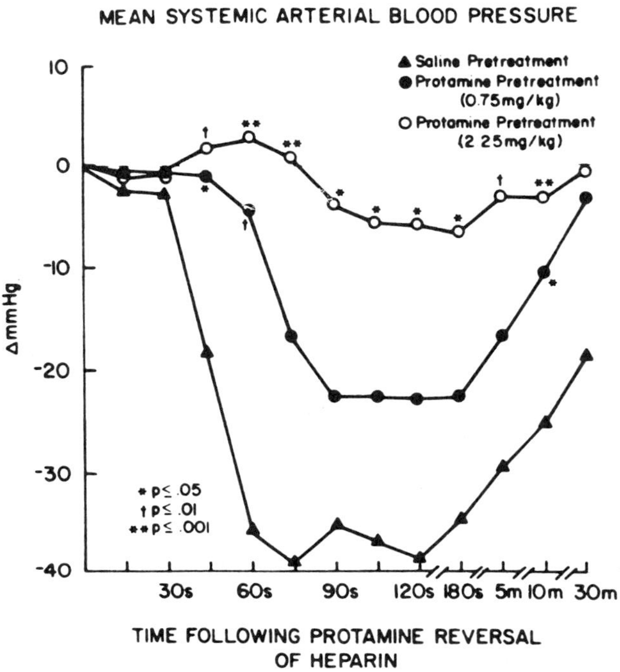

Figure 2–2. The effect of a neutralizing dose of protamine on mean systemic arterial blood pressure in two groups of dogs given protamine priming and in a control group. The curve for the control group is W-shaped, suggesting a biphasic pressure decrease. See text for implications. (From Wakefield TW, Lindblad B, Whitehouse WM, et al.: Attenuation of hemodynamic and hematologic effects of heparin-protamine sulfate interaction after aortic reconstruction in a canine model. Surgery 100:45–51, 1986.)

timing of the bradycardia and pulmonary hypertension coincided with a decrease in platelet count to 24 per cent of its initial level.

Clinical trials of the pretreatment scheme have confirmed its utility.[106] Seven patients undergoing aortic surgery received 0.75 mg•kg^{-1} of protamine 5 minutes prior to 150 units•kg^{-1} of heparin. Compared with a saline group (with proper blinding), the pretreated group experienced less systemic hypotension (+6 mm Hg maximal change vs. −16 mm Hg), less decrease in pulmonary artery pressure (+1 mm Hg vs. −7 mm Hg), and less decrease in pulmonary vascular resistance (+12 per cent vs. −15 per cent). Note that the pulmonary vascular changes in patients are opposite to those in dogs—pressure and resistance decrease instead of increase.

As with the muscle relaxant priming principle, the salutary effects of priming with protamine are not without risk. The pretreatment dose of protamine alone decreased systemic blood pressure by 14 mm Hg, almost as much as the 16 mm Hg drop seen with the neutralizing dose in the saline group. In addition, five of the seven primed patients needed additional heparin during surgery. While protamine is thought to disappear from the vasculature soon after its administration,[10] it is unlikely to be gone within a few minutes. Thus, pretreatment with protamine seems to neutralize part of the subsequently administered heparin. This explains the need for additional heparin in both the dog and the human studies. The protamine-heparin complexes formed from interaction of the priming dose of protamine and subsequent heparin probably "discharge" some of the stored mediators. This would explain the decrease in systemic blood pressure seen with the priming dose. With a partially discharged system, it is no wonder that subsequent heparin-neutralizing doses result in a tamed hemodynamic response.

Wakefield's pretreatment regimen was investigated in animals and patients undergoing aortic surgery. Would this approach work in patients undergoing CPB? Bypass patients receive larger doses of heparin and protamine. Extracorporeal circulation, hypothermia, and nonpulsatile flow induce major alterations in blood elements, in the complement system,[107, 108] and in circulating hormones.[109] If and when priming is shown to be of benefit in attenuating adverse protamine responses following bypass, the technique would need to be refined. One wonders if pretreatment can be refined, much as the priming principle for neuromuscular relaxants has been refined.[110] It needs to be determined how far in advance of heparin the protamine dose can be given, and how little can be given. Schema used to optimize the "pretreatment principle" could employ as an end point minimal changes in hemodynamics with both the priming dose and the subsequent heparin-neutralizing dose. No data are currently available to address this issue.

ALTERNATIVES TO PROTAMINE

One way to avoid adverse reactions to protamine is to eliminate its use. This goal may be approached in four general ways: first, by eliminating the need for anticoagulation during bypass; second, by anticoagulating with preparations that do not require neutralization with protamine; third, by allowing heparin activity to terminate without neutralization; and fourth, by neutralizing heparin's action with agents other than protamine. These will be considered in turn.

Construction of bypass circuits with materials that do not activate platelets or the coagulation cascade brings the promise of achieving extracorporeal circulation without the need for the large doses of heparin (300 units•kg^{-1}) now required.[111, 112] Invention of a nonthrombogenic synthetic surface would indeed be miraculous, considering the complex functions of the endothelial surface cell that it would need to mimic.[113] However, even if such a material were devised for CPB, manipulation of the vascular system for cannulation might still dictate use of moderate levels of anticoagulation (70 units•kg^{-1} of heparin); protamine would still be required for many of these patients, much as it is in the current practice of peripheral vascular surgery. While elimination of the need for anticoagulation would surely obviate the need for protamine, this goal is not likely to be achieved by advances in the field of biomaterials alone.

A second approach to avoiding the need for protamine is to anticoagulate with nonheparin preparations. Ancrod is an enzyme found in the venom of the Malayan pit viper, *Agkistrodon rhodostoma*. It anticoagulates by destroying fibrinogen. Compared with dogs given heparin, dogs given ancrod had less capillary bleeding and less deposition of platelets in their lungs and on bypass oxygenator membranes.[114] Ancrod has been used to provide anticoagulation for bypass in 20 patients.[115] Since all currently used tests of anticoagulation (ACT, PT, PTT, thrombin time) depend on the presence of fibrinogen, these tests are useless in determining the adequacy of ancrod therapy; blood fibrinogen levels are needed to monitor and assure ancrod's effectiveness. In their series, Zulys et al. initially re-established adequate coagulation by administering fresh frozen plasma (FFP) or cryoprecipitate (CP); these fluids replenished fibrinogen levels. After additional experience with this technique, they found it unnecessary to use these blood products.[115] Snake venom holds promise as an alternative to heparin for anticoagulation. Its advantages include not only avoidance of protamine, but also avoidance of the possibility of heparin-induced thrombocytopenia, and possibly improvement of blood flow across stenotic vessels owing to decreased blood viscosity from defibrinogenation. Unfortunately, the long preparation time ($>$ 12 hours) limits the usefulness of this technique.

The third alternative is to allow heparin's action to terminate spontaneously, without benefit of neutralization. In 1966, Castaneda, using "meticulous hemostasis," reported success with this technique in 92 patients.[116] He administered smaller doses of heparin than currently in use (2.0 mg•kg^{-1} with an additional 0.8 mg•kg^{-1} added to the pump prime). In addition, he did not report the use of hypothermia on CPB; heparin degradation would have been slowed at lower temperatures. Thus, for several reasons, Castaneda's patients would have had lower circulating concentrations of heparin post-bypass than those of the vast majority of patients undergoing CPB using current techniques. Yet, the patients bled considerably. Average chest tube drainage was 14.5 ml•kg^{-1} in the first 24 hours and 5.4 ml•kg^{-1} during the second 24-hour period, with a range of 1.2 to 38.3 ml•kg^{-1} in the first 24-hour period, or as much as 2.7 liters for a 70-kg person. Although Castaneda did not report requirements of blood products, it appears that common use of this technique would increase blood product use, along with an increased risk for hepatitis and acquired immune deficiency syndrome (AIDS). It is also likely that the "meticulous hemostasis" needed with this scheme might result in an increased duration of anesthesia and surgery, which has deleterious effects on patient care and health care costs.

While spontaneous decay of heparin's effect may not be a good option for routine cases, it has been reported in patients with known protamine sensitivity who require extracorporeal circulation.[104] A patient who sustained adverse cardiovascular responses to protamine during cardiac catheterization received no protamine. She bled about 5 liters over the next 13 hours and received over 15 units of blood products.

A fourth alternative to protamine is to neutralize heparin's action with substitute drugs or methods. Heparinase, an enzyme that degrades heparin, may be bonded to the exit filter of the bypass pump and used at the conclusion of bypass. Preliminary in vitro studies show that blood heparin concentrations are rapidly decreased with two passes of blood through a heparinase-bonded filter.[117] Blood flowed six times through the filter without clotting. Further research in animals on bypass is needed to determine the worthiness of this approach.

Walker et al. reasoned that platelet concentrate could neutralize heparin activity owing to the potent antiheparin activity of platelet factor 4. Two patients with a history of protamine allergy received platelet concentrate in lieu of protamine.[61] FFP (400 ml) and platelets (18 units) were given to the first patient, who bled 4 liters. The second patient received 1100 ml of FFP and 12 units of platelet concentrate; he bled 2075 ml and required exploration for bleeding 45 minutes after initial chest closure. These results are similar to those of Castaneda, who permitted spontaneous decay of heparin activity.

Toluidine blue is one of a number of alkaline dyes that bind to heparin; administration of 5 mg•kg^{-1} to dogs[16] resulted in methemoglobinemia, cyanosis, and tissue hypoxia. Smaller doses, although not toxic, did not

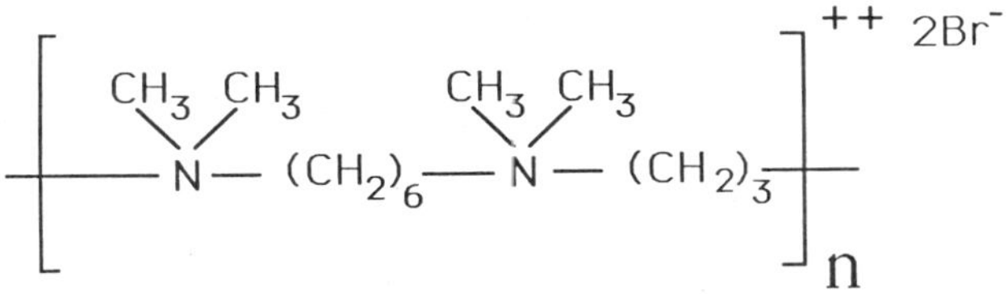

Figure 2–3. A schematic representation of the hexadimethrine molecule. The two quaternary nitrogen atoms in the repeating sequence each provide a positive charge, accounting for the polycationic properties of the polymer.

TABLE 2–4. SOME APPROACHES TO AVOIDING PROTAMINE REACTIONS

Those Attempted Clinically:
1. Slow, dilute infusion
2. Left-sided injection
3. Prophylaxis with antihistamines and/or steroids
4. Pretreatment (priming) with protamine
5. Spontaneous decay of heparin activity
6. Use of platelet concentrates to restore coagulation
Those Not in Clinical Use Today:
1. Heparinase
2. Hexadimethrine
3. Defibrinogenation (snake venom)
4. Use of nonthrombogenic synthetic materials

reduce the Lee-White WBCT sufficiently to be useful in neutralizing heparin. Quinine and benzidine have proved equally useless.[6]

Hexadimethrine (Fig. 2–3) is a synthetic polycationic compound that has been successfully used as a protamine substitute in laboratory animals and humans. It is more potent than protamine; 0.7 to 0.9 mg of hexadimethrine neutralizes 100 units of heparin compared with 1.0 to 1.4 mg of protamine.[16, 118] Compared with the heparin-protamine complex in vitro, the heparin-hexadimethrine complex is less globular, less sticky, and less stable in concentrated salt solutions.[17] Like protamine, however, rapid administration of hexadimethrine causes systemic hypotension, decreased systemic vascular resistance, and signs of histamine release.[16, 119, 120] In dogs, increases in pulmonary artery pressure accompany rapid injection of hexadimethrine only if preceded by heparin; features identical to those of protamine.[119] In addition, like protamine, hexadimethrine disappears rapidly from plasma after intravenous injection and is unavailable for neutralization of subsequently administrated heparin.[17]

While the adverse cardiovascular effects of hexadimethrine have not been linked to histamine release, complement activation, or release of thromboxane, further research of this drug would probably prove this link. Thus, hexadimethrine would most likely not be useful in avoiding type I (histamine release) and type III (pulmonary vasoconstriction) reactions. It has promise in patients who demonstrate antibodies to the protamine molecule; however, cross-reactivity between protamine and hexadimethrine is quite possible and may negate any such advantage of hexadimethrine. It is noteworthy that successful use of hexadimethrine in protamine-sensitive patients has been recently reported.[68] Hexadimethrine was withdrawn from use in the United States because of renal toxicity and difficulties in producing a polymer of appropriate molecular weight.[121, 122]

It is unfortunate that despite what appears to be a great number of approaches to avoiding protamine reactions (Table 2–4), none is sufficiently available and safe enough to be recommended strongly. Elimination of protamine toxicity will be achieved by progress along two lines. First, prospective studies must be performed to determine the incidence and the mechanism of each type of adverse response to protamine. Second, alternatives to protamine must be further developed and refined to meet clinical specifications and needs. Currently, protamine is both necessary and evil, but it need not be either.

References

1. Ando T, Yamasaki M, Suzuki K: Protamines. *In* Kleinzeller A, Springer GF, Wittmann HG (eds): Molecular Biology Biochemistry and Biophysics. Vol 12. Berlin, Springer-Verlag, 1973, pp 1–30.
2. Hagedorn HC, Jensen BN, Krarup NB, Wodstrup I: Protamine insulinate. JAMA 106:177–180, 1936.
3. Larner J: Insulin and oral hypoglycemic drugs: Glucagon. *In* Gilman AG, Goodman LS, Rall TW, Murad F (eds): The Pharmacologic Basis of Therapeutics (7th ed). New York, Macmillan, 1985, pp 1501–1502.
4. Jaques LB: Personal communication.
5. Chargaff E, Olson KB: Studies on the chemistry of blood coagulation, part VI. J Biol Chem 122:153–167, 1937–1938.
6. Jorpes E, Edman P, Thaning T: Neutralization of action of heparin by protamine. Lancet 2:975–976, 1939.
7. Jaques LB: Protamine—antagonist to heparin. J Can Med Assoc 108:1291–1297, 1973.
8. Hurt R, Perkins HA, Osborn JJ, Gerbode F: Neutralization of herpain by protamine in extracorporeal circulation. J Thoracic Surg 32:612–619, 1956.
9. Walther G, Ammon R: Anaphylaktischer shock nach protamin. Klin Wochenschr 18:288, 1939.
10. Jaques LB: A study of the toxicity of the protamine, salmine. Br J Pharmacol 4:135–144, 1949.
11. Folkman J, Langer R, Linhardt RJ, et al.: Angiogenesis inhibition and tumor regression caused by heparin or a heparin fragment in the presence of cortisone. Science 221:719–725, 1983.
12. Taylor S, Folkman J: Protamine is an inhibitor of angiogenesis. Nature 297:307–312, 1982.
13. Wright JEC: Clinical trial of protamine in the treatment of malignant diseases. Br J Cancer 22:415–421, 1968.
14. Glass DD: Management of blood and coagulation. *In* Kaplan JA (ed): Cardiac Anesthesia. Vol 2: Cardiovascular Pharmacology. New York, Grune and Stratton, 1983, pp 449–451.
15. Cobel-Geard RJ, Hassouna HI: Interaction of protamine sulfate with thrombin. Am J Hematol 14:227–233, 1983.
16. Weiss WA, Gilman JS, Catenacci AJ, Osterberg AE: Heparin neutralization with polybrene administered intravenously. JAMA 166:603–607, 1958.
17. Godal HC: A comparison of two heparin-neutralizing agents: Protamine and polybrene. Scand J Clin Lab Invest 12:446–457, 1960.
18. Ellison N, Ominsky AJ, Wollman H: Is protamine a clinically important anticoagulant? Anesthesiology 35:621–629, 1971.
19. Rådegran K, McAshlan C: Circulatory and ventilatory effects of induced platelet aggregation and their inhibition by acetylsalicylic acid. Acta Anaesthesiol Scand 16:76–84, 1972.
20. Bjoraker DG, Ketcham TR: In vivo platelet response to clinical protamine sulfate infusion. Anesthesiology 57:A7, 1982.

21. Horrow JC: Thrombocytopenia accompanying a reaction to protamine sulfate. Can Anaesth Soc J 32:49–52, 1985.
22. Morel DR, Zapol WM, Thomas SJ, et al.: C5a and thromboxane generation associated with pulmonary vaso- and bronchoconstriction during protamine reversal of heparin. Anesthesiology 66:597–604, 1987.
23. Larach DR, Waberski W: The effect of thrombocytopenia and platelet inhibition on the activated coagulation time (ACT) in man. Anesthesiology 61:A45, 1984.
24. Ellison N, Edmunds LH, Colman RW: Platelet aggregation following heparin and protamine administration. Anesthesiology 48:65–68, 1978.
25. Ellison N, Beatty CP, Blake DR, et al.: Heparin rebound: Studies in patients and volunteers. J Thorac Cardiovasc Surg 67:723–729, 1974.
26. Guffin AV , Dunbar RW, Kaplan JA, Bland JW: Successful use of a reduced dose of protamine after cardiopulmonary bypass. Anesth Analg 55:110–113, 1976.
27. Glass DD: Plasma heparin activity and antagonism during cardiopulmonary bypass with hypothermia (discussion). Anesth Analg 56:569–570, 1977.
28. Kaul TK, Crow MJ, Rajah SM, et al.: Heparin administration during extracorporeal circulation. J Thorac Cardiovasc Surg 78:95–102, 1979.
29. Fiser WP, Read RC, Wright FE, Vecchio TJ: A randomized study of beef lung and pork mucosal heparin in cardiac surgery. Ann Thorac Surg 35:615–620, 1983.
30. Racanelli A, Fareed J, Walenga JM, Coyne E: Biochemical and pharmacologic studies on the protamine interactions with heparin, its fractions and fragments. Semin Thromb Hemost 11:176–189, 1985.
31. Tinker JH, Roberts SL: Management of cardiopulmonary bypass. *In* Kaplan JA (ed): Cardiac Anesthesia (ed 2). New York, Grune and Stratton, 1987, pp 914–916.
32. Cohen JA, Frederickson EL, Kaplan JA: Plasma heparin activity and antagonism during cardiopulmonary bypass with hypothermia. Anesth Analg 56:564–570, 1977.
33. Bull BS, Huse WM, Brauer FS, Korpman RA: Heparin therapy during extracorporeal circulation. J Thorac Cardiovasc Surg 69:685–689, 1975.
34. Shapira N, Schaff HV, Piehler JM, et al.: Cardiovascular effects of protamine sulfate in man. J Thorac Cardiovasc Surg 84:505–514, 1982.
35. Frater RWM, Oka Y, Hong Y, et al.: Protamine-induced circulatory changes. J Thorac Cardiovasc Surg 87:687–692, 1984.
36. Milne B, Rogers K, Cervenko F, Salerno T: The haemodynamic effects of intraaortic versus intravenous administration of protamine for reversal of heparin in man. Can Anaesth Soc J 30:347–351, 1983.
37. Pauca AL, Graham JE, Hudspeth AS: Hemodynamic effects of intraaortic administration of protamine. Ann Thorac Surg 35:637–642, 1984.
38. Schnitzler S, Renner H, Pfuller U: Histamine release from rat mast cells induced by protamine sulfate and polyethylene imine. Agents Actions 11:73–74, 1981.
39. Foreman JC, Lichtenstein LM: Induction of histamine secretion by polycations. Biochim Biophys Acta 629:587–603, 1980.
40. Douglas WW: Histamine and 5-hydroxytryptamine (serotonin) and their antagonists. *In* Gilman AG, Goodman LS, Rall TW, Murad F (eds): The Pharmacological Bases of Therapeutics (ed 7). New York, Macmillan, 1985, p 613.
41. Hirshman CA: Personal communication.
42. Goldman BS, Joison J, Austen WG: Cardiovascular effects of protamine sulfate. Ann Thorac Surg 7:459–471, 1969.
43. Rådegran K, Taylor GA, Olsson P: Mode of action of protamine in regard to its circulatory and respiratory side effects. Eur Surg Res 3:139–148, 1971.
44. Fadali MA, Ledbetter M, Papacostas CA, et al.: Mechanism responsible for the cardiovascular depressant effect of protamine sulfate. Ann Surg 180:232–235, 1974.
45. Marin-Neto JA, Sykes MK, Marin JLB, et al.: Effect of heparin and protamine on left ventricular performance in the dog. Cardiovasc Res 13:254–259, 1979.
46. Gourin A, Streisand RL, Greineder JK, Stuckey JH: Protamine sulfate administration and the cardiovascular system. J Thorac Cardiovasc Surg 62:193–204, 1971.
47. Gourin A, Streisand RL, Stuckey JH: Total cardiopulmonary bypass, myocardial contractility, and the administration of protamine sulfate. J Thorac Cardiovasc Surg 61:160–166, 1971.

48. Stefanizyn HJ, Novick RJ, Salerno TA: Toward a better understanding of the hemodynamic effects of protamine and heparin interaction. J Thorac Cardiovasc Surg 87:678–686, 1984.
49. Rådegran K, Drugge U, Olsson P: Pulmonary venoconstriction by induced platelet aggregation. Acta Anaesthesiol Scand 18:243–247, 1974.
50. Jastrzebski J, Hilgard P, Sykes MK: Pulmonary vasoconstriction produced by protamine and protamine-heparin complex in the isolated cat lung perfused with blood or dextran. Cardiovasc Res 9:691–696, 1975.
51. Greene CE, Higgins CB, Kelley MJ, Schmidt WS, et al.: Cardiovascular effects of protamine sulfate. Invest Radiol 16:324–329, 1981.
52. Taylor RL, Little WC, Freeman GL, et al.: Comparison of the cardiovascular effects of intravenous and intraaortic protamine in the conscious and anesthetized dog. Ann Thorac Surg 42:22–26, 1986.
53. Horrow JC: Protamine: A review of its toxicity. Anesth Analg 64:348–361, 1985.
54. Conahan TJ, Andrews RW, MacVaugh H: Cardiovascular effects of protamine sulfate in man. Anesth Analg 60:33–36, 1981.
55. Michaels IA, Barash PG: Hemodynamic changes during protamine administration. Anesth Analg 62:831–835, 1983.
56. Moorthy SS, Pond W, Rowland RG: Severe circulatory shock following protamine (an anaphylactic reaction). Anesth Analg 59:77–78, 1980.
57. Olinger GN, Becker RM, Bonchek LI: Noncardiac pulmonary edema and peripheral vascular collapse following cardiopulmonary bypass: Rare protamine reaction? Ann Thorac Surg 29:20–25, 1980.
58. Lowenstein E, Johnston WE, Lappas DG, et al.: Catastrophic pulmonary vasoconstriction associated with protamine reversal of heparin. Anesthesiology 59:470–473, 1983.
59. Kern RA, Langner PH: Protamine and allergy. JAMA 113:198–200, 1939.
60. Menk EJ: Cardiac arrest following protamine sulfate infusion during regional anesthesia. Milit Med 151:318–320, 1986.
61. Walker WS, Reid KG, Hider CF, et al.: Successful cardiopulmonary bypass in diabetics with anaphylactoid reactions to protamine. Br Heart J 52:112–114, 1984.
62. Chung F, Miles J: Cardiac arrest following protamine administration. Can Anaesth Soc J 31:314–318, 1984.
63. Vierthaler LD, Becker KE Jr: Protamine anaphylaxis. Protocols for therapy in acute reactions. J Kans Med Soc 84:454–456, 1983.
64. Holland CL, Singh AK, McMaster PRB, Fang W: Adverse reactions to protamine sulfate following cardiac surgery. Clin Cardiol 7:157–162, 1984.
65. Grant JA, Cooper JR, Arens JF, et al.: Anaphylactic reactions to protamine in insulin-dependent diabetics during cardiovascular surgery. Anesthesiology 59:A74, 1983.
66. Vontz FK, Puestow EC, Cahill DJ: Anaphylactic shock following protamine administration. Ann Surg 48:549–551, 1982.
67. Cobb CA, Fung DL: Shock due to protamine hypersensitivity. Surg Neurol 17:245–246, 1981.
68. Doolan L, McKenzie J, Parsons B, Buxton B: Protamine sulfate hypersensitivity. Anasth Intensive Care 9:147–149, 1981.
69. Sharath MD, Metzger WJ, Richerson HB, et al.: Protamine-induced fatal anaphylaxis: Prevalence of antiprotamine immunoglobulin E antibody. J Thorac Cardiovasc Surg 90:86–90, 1985.
70. Kurtz AB, Gray RS, Markand S, Nabarro JD: Circlating IgG antibody to protamine in patients treated with protamine-insulins. Diabetalogia 25:322–324, 1983.
71. Levy JH, Zaidan JR, Faraj B: Prospective evaluation of risk of protamine reactions in patients with NPH insulin-depencent diabetes. Anesth Analg 65:739–742, 1986.
72. Lakin JD, Blocker TJ, Strong DM, Yocum MW: Anaphylaxis to protamine sulfate by a complement-dependent IgG antibody. J Allergy Clin Immunol 61:102–107, 1978.
73. Stoelting RK: Allergic reactions during anesthesia. Anesth Analg 62:341–356, 1983.
74. Knape JTA, Schuller JL, de Haan P, et al.: An anaphylactic reaction to protamine in a patient allergic to fish. Anesthesiology 55:324–325, 1981.
75. Caplan SN, Berkman EM: Protamine sulfate and fish allergy (letter). N Engl J Med 295:172, 1976.

76. Levy JH, Schwieger I, Faraj B, et al.: Prospective evaluation of patients with fish allergies for anaphylaxis to protamine (abstract). 9th Annual Meeting of the Society of Cardiovascular Anesthesiologists, Palm Desert, CA, May 12, 1987, p 82.
77. Hellema HWT, Rumke P: Sperm autoantibodies as a consequence of vasectomy. Clin Exp Immunol 31:18–29, 1978.
78. Samuel T, Kolk AHJ, Rumke P, Van Lis JMJ: Autoimmunity to sperm antigens in vasectomized men. Clin Exp Immunol 21:65–74, 1975.
79. Samuel T, Kolk A: Auto-antigenicity of human protamines. *In* Lepow AH, Crozier R (es): Vasectomy: Immunologic and Pathophysiologic Effects in Animals and Man. New York, Academic Press, 1979, pp 203–222.
80. Watson RA, Ansbacher R, Barry M, et al.: Allergic reaction to protamine: A late complication of elective vasectomy? Urology 22:493–496, 1983.
81. Culliford AT, Thomas S, Spencer FC: Fulminating noncardiogenic pulmonary edema. J Thorac Cardiovasc Surg 80:868–875, 1980.
82. Frater RWM: Fulminating noncardiogenic pulmonary edema (discussion). J Thorac Cardiovasc Surg 80:868–875, 1980.
83. Shaw RC: Fulminating noncardiogenic pulmonary edema (discussion). J Thorac Cardiovasc Surg 80:868–875, 1980.
84. Braimbridge MV: Fulminating noncardiogenic pulmonary edema (discussion). J Thorac Cardiovasc Surg 80:868–875, 1980.
85. Iglesias A, Nuñez L: Pulmonary edema (letter). Ann Thorac Surg 33:304, 1982.
86. Just-Viera JO, Fischer CR, Gago O, Morris JD: Acute reaction to protamine: Its importance to surgeons. Am Surg 50:52–60, 1984.
87. Hashim SW, Harold RK, Hammond GL, et al.: Noncardiogenic pulmonary edema after cardiopulmonary bypass: An anaphylactic reaction to fresh frozen plasma. Am J Surg 147:560–564, 1984.
88. Sethna DH, Moffitt E, Gray RJ, et al.: Effects of protamine sulfate on myocardial oxygen supply and demand in patients following cardiopulmonary bypass. Anesth Analg 61:247–251, 1982.
89. Hines RL, Barash PG: Protamine: Does it alter right ventricular function? Anesth Analg 65:1271–1274, 1986.
90. Levy HJ: Anaphyactic Reactions in Anesthesia and Intensive Care. Boston, Butterworths, 1986, pp 39–43.
91. Morel DR, Skoskiewicz M, Nguyenduy T, et al.: Effect of thromboxane synthesis inhibition during anaphylaxis in sheep (abstract). Anesthesiology 65:A40, 1986.
92. Levy JH: Cardiovascular changes during anaphylactic/anaphylactoid reactions in man (abstract). 8th Annual Meeting of the Society of Cardiovascular Anesthesiologists, Montreal, April 27–30, 1986, p 70.
93. Phillips SJ, Zeff RH, Kongtahworn C: Effect of protamine sulfate after cardiopulmonary bypass (letter). J Thorac Cardiovasc Surg 85:641–642, 1983.
94. Aris A, Solanes H, Bonnin JO, et al.: Intraaortic administration of protamine: Method for heparin neutralization after cardiopulmonary bypass. Cardiovasc Dis, Bull Texas Heart Inst 8:23–28, 1981.
95. Iida Y, Tsuchiya K, Sakakibara N, Tomisawa Y: Intra-aortic administration of protamine. Kyobu Geka 35:704–705, 1982.
96. Rogers K, Milne B, Salerno TA: The hemodynamic effects of inta-aortic versus intravenous administration of protamine for reversal of heparin in pigs. J Thorac Cardiovasc Surg 85:851–855, 1983.
97. Wakefield TW, Whitehouse WM, Stanley JC: Depressed cardiovascular function and altered platelet kinetics following protamine sulfate reversal of heparin activity. J Vasc Surg 1:346–355, 1984.
98. Alaoui A: Administration of protamine through left atrium (letter). J Thorac Cardiovac Surg 90:153–154, 1985.
99. Frater RWM: Administration of protamine through left atrium (letter). J Thorac Cardiovasc Surg 90:154, 1985.
100. Cherry DA, Chiu RCJ, Wynands JE, et al.: Intra-aortic vs. intravenous administration of protamine: A prospective randomized clinical study. Surg Forum 36:238–240, 1985.

101. Casthely PA, Goodman K, Fyman PN, et al.: Hemodynamic changes after the administration of protamine. Anesth Analg 65:78–80, 1986.
102. Sugawa K: The end-systolic pressure-volume relation of the ventricle: Definition, modifications, and clinical use. Circulation 63:1223, 1981.
103. Brauer S: Thoughts on protamine toxicity (letter). Anesth Analg 64:1033, 1985.
104. Campbell FW, Goldstein MF, Atkins PC: Management of the patient with protamine hypersensitivity for cardiac surgery. Anesthesiology 61:761–764, 1984.
105. Wakefield TW, Lindblad B, Whitehouse WM Jr, et al.: Attenuation of hemodynamic and hematologic effects of heparin-protamine sulfate interaction after aortic reconstruction in a canine model. Surgery 100:45–51, 1986.
106. Wakefield TW, Handler CB, Lindblad B, et al.: Protamine pretereatment attenuation of hemodynamic and hematologic effects of heparin-protamine interaction. A prospective randomized study in human beings undergoing aortic reconstructive surgery. J Vasc Surg 3:885–889, 1986.
107. Chenoweth DE, Cooper SW, Hugli TE, et al.: Complement activation during cardiopulmonary bypass: Evidence for generation of C3a and C5a anaphylatoxins. N Engl J Med 304:497–503, 1981.
108. White JV: Complement activation during cardiopulmonary bypass (letter). N Engl J Med 305:51, 1981.
109. Bovill JG, Sebel PS, Fiolet JWT, et al.: The influence of Sufentanil on endocrine and metabolic responses to cardiac surtery. Anesth Analg 62:391–397, 1983.
110. Taboada JA, Rupp SM, Miller RD: Refining the priming principle for vecuronium during rapid-sequence induction of anesthesia. Anesthesiology 64:243–247, 1986.
111. Kolff WJ, Stellwag F: Blood at artificial organ surfaces: Progress to date as steppingstones for the future. Ann NY Acad Sci 283:443–456, 1977.
112. Mason RG: The interaction of blood hemostatic elements with artificial surfaces. Prog Hemost Thromb 1:141–164, 1972.
113. Edmunds LH: The sangreal. J Thorac Cardiovasc Surg 90:1–6, 1985.
114. Berglin E, Hansson HA, Teger-Nilsson AC, William-Olsson G: Defibrinogenation as an alternative to heparinization during prolonged extracorporeal circulation in the dog. Thromb Res 9:81–93, 1976.
115. Zulys VJ, Glynn MFX, Teasdale S, et al.: Ancrod as an alternative to heparin for anticoagulation during cardiopulmonary bypass (abstract). 9th Annual Meeting of the Society of Cardiovascular Anesthesiologists, Palm Desert, CA, May 12, 1987, p 81.
116. Castaneda AR: Must heparin be neutralized following open-heart operations? J Thorac Cardiovasc Surg 52:716–719, 1966.
117. Langer R, Linhardt RJ, Hoffberg S: An enzymatic system for removing heparin in extracorporeal therapy. Science 217:261–263, 1982.
118. Keats AS, Cooley DA, Telford J: Relative antiheperin potency of polybrene and protamine in patients undergoing extracorporeal circulation. J Thorac Cardiovasc Surg 38:362–368, 1959.
119. Egerton WS, Robinson CLN: The anti-heparin, anticoagulant and hypotensive properties of hexadimethrine and protamine. Lancet 2:635–637, 1961.
120. MacKenzie GJ, Wade JD, Davies SH, Zellos S: The circulatory effects of hexadimethrine bromide (polybrene) in dogs. Am Heart J 62:511–518, 1961.
121. Wessler S, Alexander B: A Guide to Anticoagulant Therapy. New York, American Heart Association, 1970.
122. Wright JS, Osborn JJ, Perkins HA, Gerbode F: Heparin levels during and after hypothermic perfusion. J Cardiovasc Surg 5:244–250, 1964.

CHAPTER 3

FIBRINOLYSIS: A Frequent Cause of Bleeding

ALAIN J. MARENGO-ROWE and JAMES E. LEVESON

Controversy arises in the management of a bleeding patient following cardiopulmonary bypass (CPB) surgery for many reasons. Patients who have heart surgery are a heterogeneous group. Many diseases are associated with cardiac pathology; the surgical procedures performed vary greatly. There is no consensus as to what constitutes excessive bleeding, and the pathogenesis of the bleeding is poorly understood. *Notwithstanding these difficulties, we believe that the most common cause of bleeding after heart surgery is fibrinolysis.* The diagnosis of this hemorrhagic diathesis is possible using simple laboratory tests that are readily available, thus reducing the need for blood and blood components and averting re-exploratory surgery.[1] Such an approach requires excellent cooperation among all members of the team involved in the management of the patient, including nursing and laboratory personnel. While infectious diseases transmitted by transfusion have always been of concern, the increasing incidence of acquired immune deficiency syndrome (AIDS) in the general population places a great demand on therapeutic approaches that reduce blood and blood component utilization. We, therefore, describe numerous factors, often overlooked, that impinge on blood consumption and that might explain some of the very divergent opinions on the pathogenesis of the coagulopathy.

PROCEDURAL FACTORS AFFECTING BLOOD LOSS

Patients presenting for surgery vary considerably from one institution to another. Private institutions usually deal with patients from socioeconomic groups different from those of patients treated at public hospitals.

For example, Derman et al.[2] included in their small series a patient suffering from a gunshot wound to the heart. Such cases may rarely be seen in some institutions. In addition, the general health of the patient influences the outcome of surgery. A diabetic patient with coronary heart disease is clearly a different proposition than a child with cyanotic heart disease. The elderly, with reduced bone marrow and other organ reserves, must also be given special consideration, while polycythemic patients may have unusual clotting profiles.

The type of operation, whether it is on the heart or in the heart, affects both the likelihood of bleeding and the average blood loss of each patient. Bypass grafting has less effect on the hemostatic mechanism than valve replacement, which in turn differs from those surgical procedures involving aneurysms. Verska et al.[3] found that in a series of 112 patients involving 14 different surgical procedures, blood loss varied from 7.5 ml/hr/square meter of body surface area for aortic valvuloplasties to 46.2 ml/hr/square meter for double valve procedures. The duration of the operation affects not only morbidity and mortality but also the amount of hemorrhage experienced by the patient. Verska et al.[3] found blood loss to vary from 14.8 ml/hr/square meter body surface area for bypass surgery lasting less than 30 minutes to 48.3 ml/hr/square meter for operations in which bypass lasted longer than 2 hours.

The manual dexterity and experience of the surgeon performing a particular procedure also have an impact on blood loss. Yeh et al.,[4] in a series of 240 patients, compared the first 60 patients operated on with the last 60, and found that in the last 60 patients, blood loss decreased 50 per cent and blood consumption 33 per cent. The decrease was attributed to the increased experience of the surgical team. One situation in which this factor may have been overlooked (indicating some of the apparent discrepancies that can occur in the literature), is found in the report by Verska,[5] who discussed the application of the Hemochron for the control of heparin. In a sequential study involving a total of 172 patients, patients were divided into two groups. The first group of 114 patients were heparinized using a standard heparin-protamine protocol. A second group of 58 patients were controlled according to the automated activated coagulation time measured by the Hemochron. They found that blood loss was 226 ml in the early group and 153 ml in the later group. Although the investigators attributed this reduction in blood loss to better control of intraoperative heparin anticoagulation, this difference could have been due to the increased experience of the operating team. The percentage reduction in blood loss described exactly parallels the decreased blood loss noted by Yeh et al.[4] Our experience is at variance with Verska's observations. In a series of 774 patients, we observed only three patients with hemorrhage associated with heparin rebound.[6] However, as our thoracic surgical staff is increased with trainees from centers that had adopted the use of the Hemochron, we now see heparin rebound almost weekly.

Technical advances also have an effect on blood loss and can often compensate for other factors. Van Oeveren et al.[7] showed that membrane oxygenators are less traumatic to blood cells than bubble oxygenators. This concurs with earlier studies by Peterson et al.,[8] which determined that fewer platelets are sequestered in membrane oxygenators than in bubble oxygenators. The studies by Hope et al.[9] showed that the bubble oxygenator sequestered an appreciable proportion of indium-labelled platelets. Clearly, surgeons who use the membrane oxygenator will encounter fewer derangements of blood parameters in their patients.

DEFINITION OF BLEEDING

There is no universally accepted definition of what constitutes excessive bleeding. In our studies, excessive blood loss was defined as chest-tube drainage exceeding 600 ml in the first eight hours following the operation. We have now revised this definition to 200 ml or more in one hour, or 100 ml/hr for a period of at least two hours. Mohr et al.[10] define as "bleeders" a group of patients in whom closure of the sternum was delayed owing to hemorrhage. Verska et al.[3] state that a blood loss exceeding 150 ml/hr/square meter of body surface area is considered to be excessive, while in an extensive study of 512 patients, Bachmann et al.[11] considered excessive a blood loss greater than 400 ml during the first two hours following surgery. Perhaps the most stringent definition of excessive bleeding in the literature is that described by Saleem et al.,[12] who define it as greater than 100 ml in any one hour. In their series of 69 patients, there were only 20 patients who did not experience excessive bleeding. Blood consumption is often used as an indication of hemorrhage. For example, patients who required transfusion with more than 10 units of blood were classified as bleeders by Harker et al.[13] However, we feel that this is an indirect assessment of blood loss and not clinically useful. It is important to describe criteria by which the physician who is managing the patient in the immediate postoperative period can objectively decide whether to re-explore the patient or to order laboratory tests, in order to search for a coagulopathy that can be medically treated. Since the definition of excessive bleeding will vary from institution to institution, each should establish guidelines based on its own experience. In the absence of appropriate guidelines, we would agree with the observations made by Jobes and Ellison in Chapter 13, that the extensive study reported by Kirklin and Barratt-Boyes is an excellent starting point.

PATHOGENESIS OF BLEEDING

No consensus exists for the pathogenesis of nonsurgical bleeding. There are several reasons for this: There is a failure to recognize the limitations of laboratory tests; there are shortcomings in the current concepts of hemostasis; and the investigative approach is often inappropriate.

Laboratory Tests—Some Pitfalls

In order to understand the pitfalls in laboratory testing of clotting function, one must appreciate its history and pay attention to the surveys that are being performed by the College of American Pathology, which is striving to achieve consistency of data among laboratories. Also, there is a large gap between the biochemist, who is studying the structure and chemistry of blood coagulation proteins, and the practicing physician, who interprets the tests. There are few scientists and pathologists with sufficient knowledge in kinetics and protein chemistry working in hematology laboratories who can investigate the limitations of these tests. Much of the appropriate literature does not receive the attention it deserves. For example, in most laboratories today, fibrinogen is determined by a kinetic method that measures the rate of clotting of the patient's plasma in a modified thrombin clotting time. This clotting time is read on a curve using a fibrinogen standardized plasma and converted to fibrinogen concentration. However, the rate of clotting of fibrinogen is affected by both its chemical nature and its concentration. Lipinska et al.[14] isolated two forms of fibrinogen from normal plasma and prepared solutions of each form containing identical concentrations and measured their thrombin clotting times. They found that at identical concentrations, one form of fibrinogen had a thrombin clotting time of 29 seconds, while the second form had a clotting time of 41 seconds. More recently, three fibrinogens, differing in molecular weight and rate of clotting in the thrombin time (TT) test, were isolated from fresh citrated human plasma by Holm et al.[15] The differences are due to the number of carbohydrate side chains attached to the fibrinogen molecule. Plasmas from patients with liver disease have been shown to have a prolonged TT, even though their fibrinogen levels, when measured gravimetrically, are normal. In these plasmas, the fibrinogen had an additional carbohydrate chain that caused the fibrinogen to clot more slowly.[16]

The significance of these observations is that fibrinogen levels are accurate only if one assumes that the patient's plasma has the same ratio of the different forms of fibrinogen as standard plasma. This assumption, which is scientifically unwarranted, is clinically acceptable, because the alternative would be to use assays that either take too long to perform or suffer similar unwarranted assumptions. Thus, it is entirely possible that postoperative patients may release fibrinogens deficient in carbohydrates, which would clot faster and, therefore, be assessed as within normal limits, whereas in reality the actual concentration of fibrinogen is decreased. The degree of glycosylation is known to vary; this can give rise to falsely elevated estimates of fibrinogen in some patients, whereas in other patients it results in low estimates. This may explain the "compensated fibrinolysis" discussed later in the chapter.

Factor assays are also affected by the method used for their assessment. Factor assays normally involve the preparation of a standard curve, which is obtained by making a series of dilutions in buffer of an appropriate standardized plasma. Suitable commercial standards have only recently become available. We believe a similar dilution curve should always be performed on the patient's plasma in order to eliminate the possibility that interfering substances may cause erroneous estimates of factor levels. At low dilutions of plasma (1:5), these substances may cause either a shortening of the clotting time, or more often, a prolongation. At higher dilutions, the clotting times of the patient's plasma approach those of the standard plasma, thus showing that some substance is interfering with the assay. This effect is not uncommon in plasmas obtained from patients following cardiac surgery. Currently there are available two instruments that perform factor assays at a single dilution of the patient's plasma which do not show the presence of these interfering substances. This phenomenon is often seen in the postoperative period and may be caused by protamine-heparin complexes or by similar components found transiently in the patient's blood.

Other tests frequently described in the literature involve studies of various fibrin or fibrinogen fragments in plasma (fibrin[ogen] degradation products [FDP's], fibrinopeptides). They all involve some fractionation step that, by definition and not necessarily by experimental fact, establishes what one is examining. For example, Merskey et al.[17] developed the first test for FDP's but they failed in their attempts to rename this test serum fibrinogen-related antigen. Yet this description is accurate. Serum (prepared from a clot tube) is tested for antigens that are also present on fibrinogen. This test is not performed on plasma (material prepared from a tube containing anticoagulant), because fibrinogen would interfere. Since the sample is usually clotted with excess thrombin, in the presence of protamine to neutralize any heparin in the patient's sample, this test does not detect fibrinogen/fibrin fragments that coprecipitate with fibrin. Such limitations also affect many other tests performed in the laboratory. Without a knowledge of these limitations, one should be cautious in theorizing about the pathogenesis of hemorrhage.

Concepts of Hemostasis—Some Deficiencies

Much is written about hemostasis. However, there are many simple questions that one cannot answer based on current theory. Why do hemophiliacs bleed when they have a perfectly normal extrinsic coagulation mechanism? If hemophiliacs bleed because of a deficiency in clotting factor, why did Mr. Hageman not bleed, since he had a severe deficiency of an intrinsic clotting factor (Factor XII)? Why do patients with a lupus anticoagulant tend to thrombose rather than bleed, despite their prolonged activated partial thromboplastin time (aPTT)? Why do some Factor X–deficient patients have a normal aPTT and an abnormal prothrombin time (PT), and yet still suffer from hemorrhagic episodes?[18, 19] Why is Factor VII a better activator of Factor IX than its "normal activator," Factor XI? What is the basis for the concept of primary and secondary fibrinolysis? One could go on. Returning to bleeding problems following cardiac surgery, could there be a state in which blood coagulation and platelet sequestration occur in the oxygenator, while the products from this process trigger fibrinolysis in the patient? Although such a condition is clearly secondary fibrinolysis, it must be treated as primary fibrinolysis because the stimulus for it occurs extracorporeally. Clearly, much of our thinking about hemostatic mechanisms may be flawed at this time.

Investigative Approach

The prudent investigator realizes that he is studying the causes of hemorrhage following heart surgery, not the derangements of laboratory tests that may be detected as a result of cardiac surgery. This is important because one needs to know which tests will be the most valuable in the management of the bleeding patient. For this reason, the interpretation of laboratory data following surgery should be based not on what is normal in the general population but on what is normal for patients who have undergone this procedure without excessive bleeding. Tests of hemostasis should be used if they distinguish those patients who bleed from those who do not bleed excessively following cardiac surgery. Since not all patients bleed, clearly an "abnormality" seen in all patients following surgery does not explain hemorrhage. If one performs tests only on patients who bleed, it is not possible to decide if the results are a reflection of the hemorrhage or if they are deranged as a result of the procedure. Moriau et al.[20] allude to this by referring to "biological disorders," which occur in 65 per cent of their patients. These biological disorders were derangements of tests of hemostasis not associated with hemorrhage. In only 3 to 5 per cent of these patients were the disorders associated with hemorrhage. The abnormalities found in patients with biological disorders were thrombocytopenia, primary fibrinolysis, defects in coagulation, and incorrect neutralization of heparin. Mammen et al.[21] stated that since CPB introduced several changes in the hemostasis system that could be normal for a patient coming off bypass, accurate diagnosis and treatment of the bleeding problems associated with cardiac surgery can be challenging. Stated simply, a prolonged aPTT does not mean that the patient will bleed.

DO PLATELETS HAVE A ROLE?

In a detailed study, Harker et al.[13] attributed the hemorrhagic complications of cardiac surgery to the transient platelet dysfunction associated with selective alpha granule release. Although the series was small (31 patients), the patients were studied intensively. Twenty-one of the patients had no hemorrhagic problems; 10 required transfusion of more than 10 units of blood. Although these investigators found a significantly lower level of Factors V, VII, and VIII in the bleeding patients, they concluded that the increased bleeding time was the most significant finding. Harker's findings are in contrast to the investigation by Umlas[22] of 22 patients who had undergone bypass surgery. He found that 91 per cent of these patients had a normal or shorter than expected template bleeding time, and 8 of 10 patients with platelet counts of less than 100,000/μl had shorter template bleeding times that the normal corrected bleeding time. (The corrected bleeding time was that described by Harker and Slichter,[23] in which a formula was used to correct for the effect of thrombocytopenia.) Umlas' study clearly precluded the possibility of a qualitative defect in platelets following heart surgery. Perhaps the changes observed in these patients reflect a selective sequestration of platelets in the oxygenator, leaving impaired platelets in the circulation. Simple hemodilutional effects, one would presume, are not selective.

Furthermore, Martin et al.[24] studied a group of 26 patients in whom no significant hemorrhage occurred despite a decrease in platelet count and a rise in mean platelet volume following surgery. Mean platelet volume has been used by some authors as an indication of the proportion of young platelets and, hence, adequate platelet function.[25] Mohr et al.[10] used the mean platelet volume as a predictor of hemorrhagic diathesis in the immediate postoperative period. However, if Mohr's criteria were applied to the studies of Martin et al., one must conclude that all of the latter's patients were at risk for hemorrhage.

Eernisse et al.[26] emphasize the use of platelet transfusion to prevent the bleeding tendency following surgery for tetralogy of Fallot. They divided their pediatric patients into two groups. In the first group, albumin was used in the oxygenator priming solution, whereas in the second group, fresh frozen plasma (FFP) was substituted for the albumin solution. The second group was also treated with platelets postoperatively. There were 44 patients in the first group and 58 in the second. Mean blood loss was 50 ml in the first group and 27 ml in the second. Similarly, reoperation was reduced from 34 to 14 per cent; mortality also declined. Eernisse et al.[26] stressed that there were many uncontrolled variables in their study, including the facts that the surgical team had become more experienced, as evidenced by shorter perfusion times in the second group, and that the studies were run consecutively, not concurrently. The authors also could not resolve whether the reduction in blood loss could be attributed to platelet transfusions or to the use of FFP in the priming solution. In a series of 29 patients, Bagge et al.[27] showed that abnormal platelet function, as measured by platelet retention on glass beads, was extremely short-lived following neutralization of heparin with protamine.

In our studies of 774 patients, only eight had a platelet count of less than 40,000/μl; only three of the eight bled excessively. However, in two of these three, there were other coagulation derangements. Platelet aggregation studies were not reported because nearly all the patients studied following cardiac surgery had abnormal function, regardless of hemorrhagic tendency.

FIBRINOLYSIS—ITS ROLE

Many authors have associated fibrinolysis and disseminated coagulation with CPB surgery.[28–32] Umlas[33] concluded that the elevated level of fibrin split products that he found in most patients following cardiac surgery must arise from fibrinolysis rather than from disseminated intravascular coagulation. Umlas also concluded that the fibrin split products detected in these patients were not the cause of hemorrhage. Our data support this observation, since we did not find a significant difference in the levels of fibrin(ogen) split products in the serum of nonbleeders and bleeders. Derman et al.,[2] in a study of the fibrinolytic mechanism during and after cardiopulmonary extracorporeal circulation, observed a fall in euglobulin clot lysis time that was concomitant with a fall in the fibrinogen level measured gravimetrically. Gralnick et al.[34] observed a drop in plasminogen level that was concurrent with shortening of the euglobulin clot lysis time. In this small series of 25 patients, there was no laboratory abnormality that was a good predictor of hemorrhage. They also noted that the Factor V fell to a mean of 10 μ/dl, which they thought should be considered as a possible cause of hemorrhage. They excluded hypofibrinogenemia as a cause of bleeding on the grounds that the lowest fibrinogen measured was 120 mg/dl. This is at variance with our studies, in which we stressed that the mild reduction of the fibrinogen may be significant.[1] Furthermore, we postulated a state of compensated fibrinolysis in which the fibrinogen was essentially normal.[6] A possible explanation for the normal fibrinogen levels in light of hyperfibrinolysis was alluded to earlier concerning molecular heterogeneity of fibrinogen and its impact on assays. Another explanation may be a state in which lysis is matched by de novo synthesis of fibrinogen. Ekert et al.[35] described a patient who died from hyperfibrinolytic bleeding following the use of a membrane oxygenator. In their series of 11 patients, lysis was detected throughout bypass, as shown by fibrin plate lysis and euglobulin clot lysis. The antiplasmin level also fell during bypass, whereas plasminogen levels remained unchanged before and after bypass.

Bagge et al.[27] showed a large increase in circulating plasminogen activator and a precipitous fall in inhibitor to fibrinolysis (analyzed by clot lysis assay), with a concomitant fall in the levels of alpha$_2$-antiplasmin and other antiplasmins. Fibrinogen also dropped to approximately half its preoperative level during bypass.

Sterns and Lillehei[36] evaluated the effect of epsilon-aminocaproic acid (EACA) therapy in a series of 340 patients undergoing heart surgery, and concluded that this treatment results in significant blood loss. Brodsky et al.,[37] in their study of fibrinolysis in congenital heart disease, actually treated the patients prophylactically with EACA to block hyperfibrinolysis as measured by a decreased euglobulin clot lysis time. It is noteworthy that, although excessive fibrinolysis was detected in these patients, not all the patients had concomitant hypofibrinogenemia. The increase in circulating plasminogen activator levels during bypass was first demonstrated by Gans et al.,[38] who showed that activator activity increased throughout bypass and then declined when the patient came off bypass, with the rise in activator activity being mirrored by decreasing euglobulin clot lysis times. This observation had been reported earlier by Osborn et al.[39] and by von Kaulla and Swan.[40] Douglas et al.[41] showed that lysis occurred when the patients went on bypass. However, they cautioned that treatment with EACA should be restricted to those patients with a prolonged TT after heparin neutralization. They found a correlation between mortality and the postoperative prolongation of the TT. In addition, they noted that the percentage fall in platelet count during bypass surgery correlated with the case number in the series.

Phillips et al.[42] found that fibrinolysis was the major contributor to bleeding. However, they stressed that the activation of profibrinolysin (plasminogen) was highly significant because they thought hemorrhage was the result of the activation of profibrinolysin rather than of hypofibrinogenemia. It could be that the anoxic blood that pools in the microvasculature during anesthesia causes this fibrinolytic activity.

Strictly speaking, "fibrinolytic activity" that appears to increase may be better defined as proteolytic activity. In the laboratory, this proteolytic activity is detected by the plasma's ability to lyse fibrin. This proteolytic activity declines to very low levels within 48 hours after surgery but then rises to preoperative levels after seven days. This may be a manifestation of the disturbances of protein metabolism that Moyer et al.[43] studied in patients following surgery. They noticed that during hemorrhagic shock and massive surgery, the liver switches to utilizing amino acids as a source of energy. The liver, in making this switch, mobilizes body proteins, resulting in an increase in essential amino acids in the circulation. While most patients can control this phenomenon, the ones who cannot do so succumb to multiple organ failure. Perhaps the fibrinolysis observed in post-bypass patients is a manifestation of this process. Conversely, any patient who bleeds long enough will sooner or later develop excessive proteolytic activity. This arises as a result of the bleeding rather than as a cause of it.

An additional problem facing the physician managing bleeding patients is long laboratory turnaround times. Rapid changes can occur, not only as a result of hemorrhage, but also as a result of transfusion. Long turnaround times result in the physician's receiving test information that may no longer be relevant because the patient's status has changed. This point is emphasized when a suture line breaks. The need to obtain rapid information has caused many physicians to resort to equipment produced by companies that are marketing their latest quick-fix solution to this problem. Often the rationale for the use of a test is that it is more physiological. This is a hypothesis, not a truism, and therefore should be tested. We do not know of any physiological laboratory test.

It is our view, therefore, that the appropriate clinical management should not rely on laboratory testing alone to explain complex systems. Astute clinical judgment based on objective and time-tested assessment of successful therapy is also needed. Following major surgery, extensive proteolysis occurs with the destruction of proteins, including coagulation factors and fibrinogen. This proteolysis may be systemic, but it may also be localized, such as phagocytosis by white cells chemotactically drawn to blood clots in the chest cavity. This proteolytic process can be controlled by the use of EACA. If the coagulopathy is severe, cryoprecipitate (CP) and FFP may also be necessary to replace the destroyed coagulation factors. These blood components contain not only clotting factors but also plasminogen, which is necessary to form the plasminogen-EACA complex. It is perhaps this complex that helps to inhibit proteolytic activity. It is known tht elastase, a proteolytic enzyme that is found to be increased following surgery, degrades plasminogen so that it will no longer bind EACA.[44] FFP and CP may replace this plasminogen that, incongruously, is essential for effective EACA therapy. In an earlier publication,[6] we reported the guidelines employed by our institution for the use of EACA and blood components following cardiac surgery (Table 3–1). It is important to emphasize that this approach is applied promptly to arrest hemorrhage, because the longer a patient bleeds, the more difficult it is to arrest the hemorrhage. FFP is used to correct a prolonged PT, since this blood component contains all the clotting factors. The use of CP to correct a prolonged aPTT was adopted by clinical trial, and CP has been used extensively in our institution for this particular situation. However, studies of Factor VIII, fibrinogen, and von Willebrand factor levels have failed to explain why CP is successful in correcting a prolonged aPTT in these patients.

MANAGEMENT OF PATIENTS WHO BLEED

The management of patients with excessive hemorrhage after CPB can be difficult because of the many variables, both surgical and nonsurgical, involved. As many surgeons have found, re-exploration of these patients is frustrating because often only generalized oozing is found. Our approach to the bleeding patient is based on clinical evaluation in conjunction with a battery of simple laboratory tests that can be rapidly performed, namely PT, aPTT, fibrinogen, platelet count, TT or Tri-F-Titer, and hematocrit. Bleeding is assessed by measuring chest tube drainage from tubes that have been regularly stripped, and also by inspecting the surgical wounds. A baseline study consisting of PT, aPTT, fibrinogen, TT or Tri-F-Titer, and platelet count is performed on all patients both preoperatively and immediately postoperatively. This baseline study achieves two goals. The first is that it identifies those patients who are at increased risk of bleeding. The patients most likely to suffer from bleeding directly related to a hematological cause were those who postoperatively exhibited one or more of the hematological parameters

TABLE 3–1. CLASSIFICATION AND TREATMENT OF PATIENTS WITH EXCESSIVE POSTOPERATIVE BLEEDING

Cause of Bleeding	PT > 19 sec	PTT > 45 sec	Fibrinogen < 225 mg/dl	TFT ≤ 1 : 32	Treatment
Compensated hyperfibrinolysis	No	No	No	Yes	Amicar
Uncompensated hyperfibrinolysis	Yes/No	Yes	Yes	Yes	Amicar; cryoprecipitate; FFP
Heparin	Yes/No	Yes	No	Heparin effect	Protamine
Surgical	No	No	No	No	Re-exploration

PT = Prothrombin time; PTT = partial thromboplastin time; TFT = tri-F titer; FFP = fresh frozen plasma. (Copyright by A. J. Marengo-Rowe, M.D.)

in Table 3–2. The second is that it gives a basis for comparison should the patient start to bleed.

Increased bleeding, if hematologically generated, is usually associated with increasing derangements of the hemostatic parameters when compared with the baseline study. Repeat studies should always be used after therapy in order to establish that the hemostatic parameters have returned to normal, indicating that the hemostatic derangement has been corrected. For patients in whom very dynamic changes can occur and in whom there is increased turnover of the constituents of blood, it is not possible to assess correct dosage of blood components except by repeat testing. *It is our practice to repeat studies as necessary in the bleeding patient so that appropriate blood components are transfused in the smallest quantities needed to effect hemostasis.* Changes in test values are taken into consideration, as well as absolute and average values obtained on all patients who have undergone this procedure. For example, the PT is often prolonged following heart surgery, but prolongation beyond 19 seconds is significant in light of hemorrhage. A patient who is bleeding at 100 ml/hr may not need treatment if the tests are marginally "abnormal" and are improving. The patient who bleeds and who experiences sudden onset of hemorrhage greater than 400 ml/hr is surgically re-explored. A slower bleed, if fibrinogen is essentially normal, will be treated with EACA alone. However, if bleeding occurs concurrently with a low fibrinogen or prolonged aPTT, CP is used in conjunction with EACA. Similarly, if the PT is unusually prolonged when compared with the norm for this group of patients, FFP may also be needed. However, these measures are used only after the presence of unneutralized heparin has been excluded. Heparin may be detected by the Tri-F-Titer or the combination of the TT and reptilase times. The presence of heparin, even in low concentrations, is always significant and must be corrected. For procedures in which there has been extensive use of cardiotomy suckers, approximately 10 to 20 per cent higher blood loss is usual. In these patients, especially in the elderly with reduced bone marrow reserves and in those whose platelet count falls below 40,000/μL, platelet transfusions may be necessary. Utilizing this approach in more than 2000 adult patients, we found that excessive fibrinolysis can be successfully

TABLE 3–2. POSTOPERATIVE HEMATOLOGICAL PARAMETERS ASSOCIATED WITH INCREASED RISK OF HEMORRHAGE

PT	>19 sec
aPTT	>45 sec
Fibrinogen	<225 mg/dl
Platelets	<40 thousand/μl
Presence of unneutralized heparin	

treated with EACA (10 to 20 grams) alone or in combination with CP or FFP. This approach resulted in the mean use per patient of 2.1 units of packed red cells, 2.5 units of CP, and less than one unit of FFP and platelets per patient admission. The rates of surgical re-exploration and of infection were markedly reduced. Deep vein thrombosis and pulmonary embolus were not problems.

A final comment: It has been our experience that the mechanism proposed for the study of a disease process often is a function of the latest methodology and equipment available to the researcher. Since the techniques to study platelets have become more widely available, research has been focussed on platelets, as well as on their role in the causation of hemorrhage following heart surgery. Perhaps the discovery of the fibrinolytic factors Protein S and Protein C will bring renewed interest in fibrinolysis.

Acknowledgment

To Mrs. Hilda Goodman Roosth with affection in acknowledgment of her example, courage, and many courtesies.

References

1. Marengo-Rowe AJ, Lambert CJ, Levenson JE, et al.: The evaluation of hemorrhage in cardiac patients who have undergone extracorporeal circulation. Transfusion 19:426–433, 1979.
2. Derman UM, Rand PW, Barker N: Fibrinolysis after cardiopulmonary bypass and its relationship to fibrinogen. J Thorac Cardiovasc Surg 51:223–228, 1966.
3. Verska JJ, Lonser ER, Brewer LA III: Predisposing factors and management of hemorrhage following open heart surgery. J Cardiovasc Surg 13:361–368, 1972.
4. Yeh T Jr, Shelton L, Yeh T: Blood loss and bank blood requirement in coronary bypass surgery. Ann Thorac Surg 26:11–16, 1978.
5. Verska JJ: Control of heparinization by activated clotting time during bypass with improved postoperative hemostasis. Ann Thorac Surg 24:170–173, 1977.
6. Lambert CJ, Marengo-Rowe AJ, Levenson JE, et al.: The treatment of postperfusion bleeding using epsilon-aminocaproic acid, cryoprecipitate, fresh-frozen plasma, and protamine sulfate. Ann Thorac Surg 28:440–444, 1979.
7. van Oeveren W, Kazatchkine MD, Descamps-Latscha B, et al.: Deleterious effects of cardiopulmonary bypass: A prospective study of bubble versus membrane oxygenation. J Thorac Cardiovasc Surg 89:888–899, 1985.
8. Peterson KA, Dewanjee MK, Kaye MP: Fate of indium m-labeled platelets during cardiopulmonary bypass performed with membrane and bubble oxygenators. J Thorac Cardiovasc Surg 84:39–43, 1982.
9. Hope AF, Heyns A duP, Lotter MG, et al.: Kinetics and sites of sequestration of indium III-labeled human platelets during cardiopulmonary bypass. J Thorac Cardiovasc Surg 81:880–886, 1981.
10. Mohr R, Martinowitz U, Golan M, et al.: Platelet size and mass as an indicator for platelet transfusion after cardiopulmonary bypass. Circulation 74(Suppl 3):153–158, 1986.
11. Bachmann F, McKenna R, Cole ER, Najafi H: The hemostatic mechanism after open-

heart surgery. I. Studies on plasma coagulation factors and fibrinolysis in 512 patients after extracorporeal circulation. J Thorac Cardiovasc Surg 70:76, 1975.
12. Saleem A, Blifeld C, Saleh S, et al.: Viscoelastic measurement of clot formation: A new test of platelet function. Ann Clin Lab Sci 13:115–124, 1983.
13. Harker LA, Malpass TW, Branson HE, et al.: Mechanism of abnormal bleeding in patients undergoing cardiopulmonary bypass: Acquired transient platelet dysfunction associated with selective alpha-granule release. Blood 56:824–834, 1980.
14. Lipinska I, Lipinski B, Gurewich V: Fibrinogen heterogeneity in human plasma. Electrophoretic demonstration and characterization of two major fibrinogen components. J Lab Clin Med 84:509–516, 1974.
15. Holm B, Nilsen DWT, Kierulf P, Godal HC: Purification and characterization of 3 fibrinogens with different molecular weights obtained from normal human plasma. Thromb Res 37:165–176, 1985.
16. Gralnick HR, Givelber H, Abrams E: Dysfibrinogenemia associated with hepatoma. N Engl J Med 299:221–226, 1978.
17. Merskey C, Kleiner GJ, Johnson AJ: Quantitative estimation of split products of fibrinogen in human sera, relation to diagnosis and treatment. Blood 28:1–18, 1966.
18. Girolami A, Vicarioto G, Ruzza G, et al.: Factor X Padua: A 'new' congenital Factor X abnormality with a defect only in the extrinsic system. Acta Haematol 73:31–36, 1985.
19. Nora RE, Bell WR, Noe DA, Sholar PW: Novel Factor X deficiency. Normal partial thromboplastin time and associated spindle cell thymoma. Am J Med 79:122–125, 1985.
20. Moriau M, Masure R, Hurlet A, et al.: Haemostasis disorders in open heart surgery with extracorporeal circulation. Vox Sang 32:41–51, 1977.
21. Mammen EF, Koets MH, Washington BC, et al.: Hemostasis changes during cardiopulmonary bypass surgery. Semin Thromb Hemost 11:281–291, 1985.
22. Umlas J: In vivo platelet function following cardiopulmonary bypass. Transfusion 15:596–599, 1975.
23. Harker LA, Slichter SJ: The bleeding time as a screening test for evaluation of platelet function. N Engl J Med 287:155, 1972.
24. Martin JF, Daniel TD, Trowbridge A: Acute and chronic changes in platelet volume and count after cardiopulmonary bypass induced thrombocytopenia in man. Thromb Haemost 57:55–58, 1987.
25. Eldor A, Avitzour M, Or R, et al.: Prediction of haemorrhagic diathesis in thrombocytopenia by mean platelets volume. Br Med J 285:397–400, 1982.
26. Eernissee JG, Brand A, Repelaer van Driel OJ, Dirksen TH: Prevention of bleeding tendency after open-heart surgery for Tetralogy of Fallot. Scand J Thorac Cardiovasc Surg 11:105–109, 1977.
27. Bagge L, Lilienberg G, Nystrom SO, Tyden H: Coagulation, fibrinolysis and bleeding after open-heart surgery. Scand J Thorac Cardiovasc Surg 20:151–160, 1986.
28. Bloom AL: Activation of coagulation and fibrinogen loss after using extracorporeal circulation. J Clin Pathol 16:558, 1963.
29. Deykin D: The clinical challenge of disseminated intravascular coagulation. N Engl J Med 283:36, 1970.
30. Dutton RC, Edmunds LH Jr, Hutchinson JC, Roc BB: Platelet aggregate emboli produced in patients during cardiopulmonary bypass with membrane oxygenators and blood filters. J Thorac Surg 67:258, 1974.
31. Karpatkin M: Diagnosis and management of disseminated intravascular coagulation. Pediatr Clin North Am 18:23, 1971.
32. Penick GD, Averette HE Jr, Peters RM, Brinkhaus KM: The hemorrhagic syndrome complicating extracorporeal shunting of blood: An experimental study of its pathogenesis. Thrombo Diath Haemorrh 2:218–225, 1958.
33. Umlas J: Fibrinolysis and disseminated intravascular coagulation in open heart surgery. Transfusion 16:460–463, 1976.
34. Gralnick HR, Fischer RD: The hemostatic response to open-heart operations. J Thorac Cardiovasc Surg 61:909, 1971.
35. Ekert H, Montgomery D, Aberdeen E: Fibrinolysis during extracorporeal circulation.

Comparison of the effects of disc and membrane oxygenators. Circ Res 28:512–517, 1971.
36. Sterns LP, Lillehei CW: Effect of epsilon aminocaproic acid upon blood loss following open-heart surgery: An analysis of 340 patients. Can J Thorac Surg 36:519–530, 1958.
37. Brodsky I, Gill DN, Lusch CJ: Fibrinolysis in congenital heart disease. Am J Clin Pathol 51:51–57, 1969.
38. Gans H, Lillehei CW, Krivit W: Problems in hemostasis during open-heart surgery. I. On the release of plasminogen activator. Ann Surg 154:915–924, 1961.
39. Osborn J, Mackenzie JJR, Shaw A, et al.: Cause and prevention of hemorrhage following extracorporeal circulation. Surg Forum 6:96, 1955.
40. Von Kaulla KN, Swan H: Clotting deviations in man during cardiac bypass: Fibrinolysis and circulating anticoagulants. J Thorac Surg 36:519, 1958.
41. Douglas AS, McNicol GP, Bain WH, Mackey WA: The haemostatic defect following extracorporeal circulation. Br J Surg 53:455–467, 1966.
42. Phillips LL, Malm JR, Deterling RA: Coagulation defects following extracorporeal circulation. Ann Surg 157:317–326, 1963.
43. Moyer ED, Border JR, Cerra FB, et al.: Multiple systems organ failure. IV. Imbalances in plasma amino acids associated with exogenous albumin in the trauma-septic patient. J Trauma 21:543–547, 1981.
44. Magnussen S: Personal communication, 1983.

CHAPTER 4

FIBRINOLYTIC THERAPY

JUDITH A. FABIAN and LAURAINE STEWART

With the advent of thrombolytic therapy in the treatment of acute myocardial infarction (AMI), it was inevitable that failure of that therapy in some patients would necessitate immediate surgical correction of their coronary insufficiency. It is mandatory, therefore, that cardiac anesthesiologists have an appreciation of the chemistry and pharmacology of the fibrinolytic system and the drugs that affect it.

THE FIBRINOLYTIC ENZYME SYSTEM

The role of the fibrinolytic enzyme system in the blood is the removal of fibrin from the vascular bed. The fibrinolytic system consists of plasminogen (Pg), plasmin (Pm), activators of plasminogen, inhibitors of plasmin and plasminogen activators, and fibrinogen and fibrin.

Activators of plasminogen include streptokinase (SK), urokinase (UK), prourokinase (pro-UK), and tissue-type plasminogen activator (t-PA). Inhibitors include anti-activators (anti-SK, anti-UK, anti-t-PA) and antiplasmins, which inhibit the plasmin formed from circulating plasminogen (Fig. 4–1).

Plasminogen and Plasmin

Native human plasminogen is a single-chain glycoprotein with a molecular weight of 92,000 to 94,000 daltons. Two subforms having slightly different molecular weights and physical and chemical properties may be isolated using affinity chromatography. Glutamic acid (Glu) is the terminal amino acid for both subforms.[1]

Human plasminogen consists of 790 amino acids containing 24 disulfide bridges.[2] In addition, a portion of plasminogen can be represented

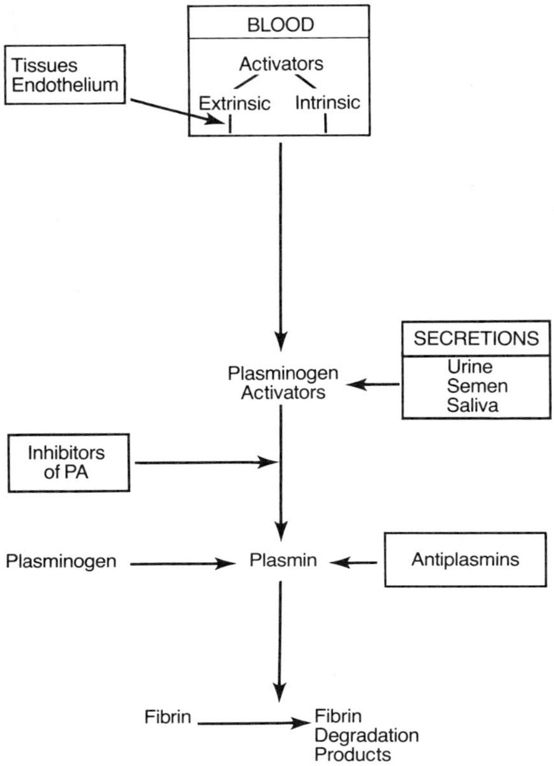

Figure 4–1. The fibrinolytic enzyme system.

by 5 "kringles," or homologous triple loop structures, with interconnecting peptide strands (Fig. 4–2).[3] Proteolytic digestion of native plasminogen yields several important lower molecular weight forms. Nomenclature of these molecules is based on the amino-terminal amino acid. Therefore, native circulating human plasminogen is referred to as Glu^1-plasminogen (Glu^1-Pg). Cleavage of Glu^1-Pg at the Lys^{76}-Lys^{77} peptide bond yields Lys^{77}-Pg,[4] which is more asymmetrical and flexible than Glu^1-Pg, and is converted to plasmin by cleavage of the Arg^{560}-Val^{561} bond.

Other low molecular weight plasminogen molecules have been isolated by limited proteolysis of Glu^1-Pg. These zymogens are all capable of activation to plasmin and probably exist as independent domains in the Lys^{77}-Pg structure.[1]

Lysine-binding sites in plasminogen mediate its interaction with fibrin, $alpha_2$-antiplasmin, and histidine-rich glycoprotein (HRGP).[5] It has been suggested that these sites play an important role in the regulation of fibrinolysis.[6]

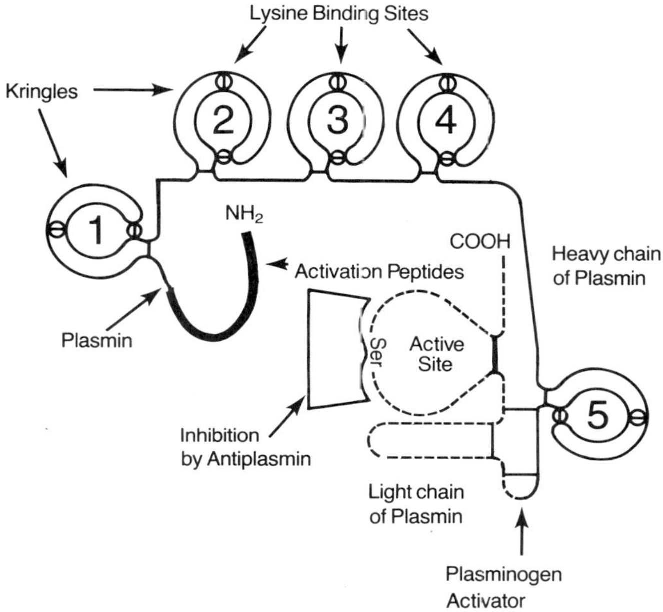

Figure 4–2. Diagram of human plasminogen. Plasminogen activators cleave the Arg^{560}-Val^{561} peptide blood (at the beginning of the dotted line). Activation peptides (heavy line) are liberated by the action of plasmin on the amino-terminal. When this occurs at Lys^{76}-Lys^{77}, Lys^{77}-Pg is left behind. The five "kringles" are located on the heavy chain. α_2-Antiplasmin reacts with the serine active site on the light chain, inhibiting protease activity. (Modified from Castellino FJ: Recent advances in the fibrinolytic system. Chem Rev 81:431–446, 1981. Copyright 1981 American Chemical Society.)

Plasmin is a two-chain molecule stabilized by two sulfide bonds. It is composed of a heavy chain called the A-chain, which originates from the NH_2-terminal portion of plasminogen, and a light chain called the B-chain, which is the COOH-terminal portion.

Native plasmin is formed by the cleavage of at least two peptide bonds in plasminogen. Plasmin nomenclature is based on the NH_2-terminal amino acid of the *heavy* chain, since all light chains have the same NH_2-terminal amino acid, Val^{561}. This is because one of the peptide cleavages must be at Arg^{560}-Val^{561} for catalytic activity to be expressed.[7]

Activation of Glu^{1}-Pg or Lys^{77}-Pg yields native plasmin, Lys^{77}-Pm. However, other plasmins such as Glu^{1}-Pm and Val^{442}-Pm are prepared in the laboratory.[1]

Assays of plasmin are based on its capability to digest many proteins (fibrin, fibrinogen, Factors V and VIII, casein), various esters, and amides. Although plasminogen has no such activity, it may be assayed after conversion to plasmin in similar systems.

Plasminogen Activators

Activators of plasminogen have been found in a variety of sources. The two most widely studied are UK and SK. Other such agents exist in blood, tissues, and secretions, but their interrelationships are only now being studied in detail.

Urokinase is a trypsin-like serine protease. It may occur in two molecular forms of differing molecular weights (high molecular weight UK: 54,000 daltons; and low molecular weight UK: 33,000 daltons). Both forms are equally active. The low molecular weight form is a degradation product of the high molecular weight form.[8] UK has been isolated from human urine and cultured human embryonic kidney cells.

Regarding possible protein substrates, the only UK substrate is plasminogen; UK activates plasminogen directly to plasmin. It is a highly specific enzyme that hydrolyzes a peptide link in plasminogen, converting it to plasmin. UK directly activates plasminogen in a dose-related fashion; i.e., the amount of plasmin produced is directly related to the concentration of UK.[9] The presence of fibrin and its metabolic products has been demonstrated to stimulate the activation of Glu^1-Pg by UK.[2]

Some success has been achieved in thrombolytic therapy with UK, but its therapeutic role has not been clearly defined. SK has gained more widespread use because experience has shown treatment to be more effective and more rapid.[10] In addition, SK is easier to obtain and is far less expensive.[2]

SK is a nonenzymatic protein with a molecular weight of 47,000 daltons. It is produced by beta-hemolytic *Streptococcus* of Lancefield group C. The only known substrates are plasminogens from plasma of humans as well as that of a number of other species.[1] Fibrin and its breakdown products have been shown to enhance plasminogen activation by SK.[11]

SK activates plasminogen in a stepwise manner. First, it binds with plasminogen to form an equimolar complex (SK-Pg). This interaction results in a conformational alteration in the complex, exposing an active site in the plasminogen moiety (SK-Pg′). the SK-Pg′ complex combines with fibrin with the same degree of affinity as plasmin. This complex is not stable; it is rapidly altered to a complex of SK and plasmin (SK-Pm). The SK-Pm complex then enzymatically converts plasminogen to plasmin (Fig. 4–3).[1, 9]

Large doses of SK will form many active complexes, with little plasminogen remaining to be activated to plasmin. Conversely, when lower doses of SK are administered, only a small amount of plasminogen will be complexed, so that large amounts of active plasmin can be produced.[10]

The presence of inhibitors of fibrinolysis must be taken into account

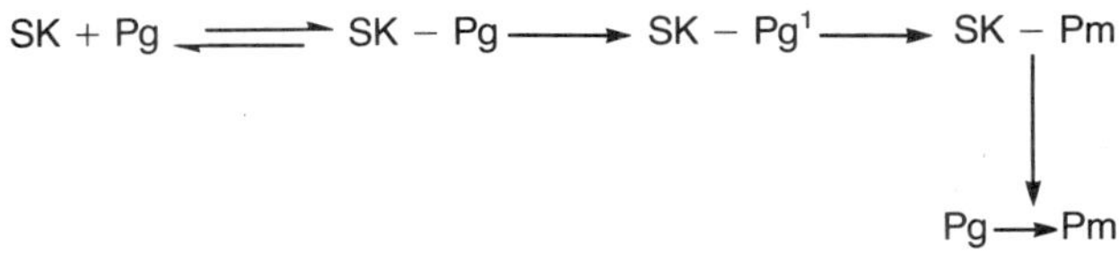

Figure 4–3. Streptokinase activation of plasminogen to plasmin.

during thrombolytic therapy. Most important is the plasmin inhibitor, alpha$_2$-antiplasmin. Other natural inhibitors include UK-inhibitor, as well as varying levels of antibodies to SK which have been acquired from previous streptococcal infections.[12] At the onset of therapy, a loading dose of SK sufficiently large to neutralize the SK antibodies is needed before fibrinolytic activation can be obtained. Furthermore, the starting dose must be high enough to overcome the barrier represented by alpha$_2$-antiplasmin.[10] Laboratory studies indicate that the levels of alpha$_2$-antiplasmin must be reduced by 60 per cent before these fibrinolytic agents are able to exert their effect.[13]

A significant risk associated with SK therapy is the possibility of a severe allergic reaction. Corticosteroids are frequently used as adjuvant therapy in an attempt to avoid this complication. After a few days of SK infusions, the anti-SK titers may rise 50 to 100 times the preinfusion levels and remain high for four to six months. During this time attempts to reinstitute therapy would be ineffective.[2]

The second, or maintenance, phase of therapy is calculated to maintain a therapeutic level of SK-Pg. The complex attaches to the surface of the clot, converting plasminogen both on the surface and in the interior to plasmin, which in turn transforms insoluble fibrin into soluble peptides. Activator complex that is not bound to the clot converts newly formed plasminogen into plasmin, which would also have a lytic effect on the clot.[10]

Free SK has no specific affinity for fibrin and indiscriminately activates both circulating and fibrin-bound plasminogen to plasmin. Alpha$_2$-antiplasmin has no effect on the SK-Pg activator complex, but circulating plasmin is almost immediately neutralized by alpha$_2$-antiplasmin. Once the inhibitor is exhausted, plasmin then digests other coagulation factors, e.g., fibrinogen, Factor V, and Factor VIII, resulting in a bleeding diathesis.[2]

Hemorrhage is the most serious risk of thrombolytic therapy. Lew and Ganz reported serious hemorrhagic complications in 13.6 per cent of their patients, with complication rates being the greatest (26 per cent) in elderly patients (>70 years).[14] Consequently, any condition that predisposes a patient to hemorrhage or any condition in which anticoagulation is contraindicated also contraindicates thrombolytic therapy. The presence of such complications has stimulated active research in the development of thrombolytic agents that preferentially activate the thrombolytic system in proximity to the fibrin clot. Such fibrin-selective agents are anticipated to have fewer side effects. Substances with the potential for satisfying these criteria include pro-UK, t-PA, and acylated plasmin-streptokinase complex (acyl-SK).

Inactive pro-UK is a glycoprotein that is the native single-chain precursor of UK. It has a molecular weight of 55,000 daltons. The single-chain proenzyme is converted to fully active two-chain UK by plasmin. The gene of human UK has been cloned and expressed in *Escherichia coli* as recombinant pro-UK, which remains stable in the absence of a fibrin clot but is slowly activated in its presence. Pro-UK has potent thrombolytic activity and better thrombus selectivity than recombinant two-chain UK. It is quickly converted to fully active UK by traces of plasmin generated through the activation of plasminogen by recombinant pro-UK.[10] If fibrin specificity is maintained at therapeutic plasma concentrations, then pro-UK has the potential for being a valuable thrombolytic agent.

Acyl enzymes are new thrombolytic agents in which the SK-Pg complex is chemically modified by the location of an acyl group in the active center of the transitory Sk-Pg′ complex. Two different compounds of Lys-Pg–acyl-SK complex, BRL 26921 and BRL 33575, are being investigated. Deacylation results in a functionally active plasminogen activator. It was anticipated that binding of the acylated complexes to fibrin, followed by deacylation, would result in the generation of fibrin-associated plasmin and, consequently, a more fibrin-specific thrombolytic effect. It has been reported, however, in preliminary studies using therapeutic levels of BRL 26921 followed by maintenance injections, that a defibrination syndrome was observed.[15]

T-PA is a serine protease with a molecular weight of about 70,000 daltons. It is converted into a two-chain molecule linked to plasmin by a disulfide bridge. Single- and double-chain forms have similar fibrinolytic and plasminogen-activating properties.[15]

The first pure form of human t-PA was obtained from the uterus. Using an antiserum derived from this preparation, it has been shown that tissue, vascular, and blood plasminogen are immunologically identical to one another but different from UK. T-PA has been harvested from the culture medium of human melanoma cells, and the human t-PA gene has been cloned and expressed.[15]

In the presence of fibrin, t-PA has a high affinity for plasminogen. Effective in vivo thrombolysis appears to be regulated by the adsorption of t-PA and plasminogen to the surface of fibrin, resulting in the local production of plasmin. Plasmin formed on the fibrin surface is slowly inactivated by alpha$_2$-antiplasmin. The fibrinolytic process is therefore initiated by fibrin and is confined to its surface. Limited experience involving studies in humans suggests that specific thrombolysis without systemic activation of the fibrinolytic system can be achieved with t-PA.[15]

Inhibitors of Fibrinolysis

Several protease inhibitors capable of neutralizing plasmin exist in plasma. The major one is a protein with a molecular weight of 60,000 to 70,000 daltons known as alpha$_2$-antiplasmin.[16] It rapidly forms a reversible complex with Lys^{77}-Pm, which then converts to an irreversible complex. This interaction is influenced by the availability of lysine-binding sites on plasmin. If the ability of alpha$_2$-antiplasmin to bind with plasmin is overwhelmed, then alpha$_2$-macroglobin may act as a reserve of antiplasmin activity. Other proteins have minor roles as physiological antiplasmins. Isolated deficiency of alpha$_2$-antiplasmin results in a severe bleeding disorder, whereas deficiency of the other antiplasmins does not.[17]

Inhibitors of both t-PA and UK have been isolated from endothelial cell cultures as well as from platelets and placenta. These inhibitors have extremely rapid action kinetics. Plasma concentrations are very low, but increases of 10 to 20 times have been described in certain thrombotic conditions.[12]

Epsilon-aminocaproic acid (EACA) and its analogues are well known to produce in vivo antifibrinolytic effects. Studies reveal that EACA induces striking conformational alterations in molecules possessing the amino-terminal peptide Glu^1-Lys,^{76} including Glu^1-Pg. However, molecules such as Lys^{77}-Pg, which do not contain this peptide, do not undergo such a conformational change even though they are capable of binding EACA.[18] Trans-4-(aminomethyl)cyclohexane-1-carboxylic acid (t-AMCHA or transexamic acid) produces the same alterations; potency is increased by the interposition of the cyclohexane ring.

Studies indicate that EACA and its analogues interact with the latent heavy plasmin chain of plasminogen, generating a more asymmetrical and internally flexible form of the protein.[1] It also appears that the site of interaction of EACA and its analogues with plasminogen is at the kringles. There exists a strong binding site for EACA on Kringle 1 (K1); the five weaker binding sites are on the other kringles.

In lower concentrations in vitro, EACA enhances the activation of Glu^1-Pg by UK; increasing the EACA concentration in the activation mixture results in inhibition in the presence of UK. Why the initial enhancement does not result in an in vivo fibrinolytic effect is not clear. However, it appears that at low concentrations, the action of EACA and its analogues is to displace plasmin(ogen) from fibrin, and this involves the strong EACA site in plasminogen. At slightly higher EACA concentrations affecting the weak binding sites, the activation of Glu[1]-Pg[1] is enhanced, but a fibrinolytic effect does not result, since this activation takes place *away* from the fibrin strand. At higher concentrations of EACA, plasmin and UK activity are inhibited.[1]

FIBRINOLYSIS

The balance that allows fibrinolysis to occur on a local basis only depends on two factors: (1) the affinity of formed fibrin and plasminogen activators and (2) the opposing affinity of plasma alpha$_2$-antiplasmin for free plasmin.[19]

Native fibrinogen (molecular weight of 343,000 daltons) is composed of three pairs of nonidentical peptide chains ($A\alpha^2$, $B\beta^2$, γ^2) stabilized by disulfide bonds. To accomplish the conversion of fibrinogen to fibrin, thrombin catalyzes cleavage of fibrinopeptides A and B from the $A\alpha$ and $B\beta$ chans, yielding the α and β chains of the fibrin monomer, which polymerizes to yield a form of fibrin. Thrombin then catalyzes the activation of fibrin-stabilizing factor (Factor XIII), which catalyzes the formation of intermolecular crosslinks between the γ chains (forming γ-γ dimers) and between the α chains (forming α-α multimers).[1]

Small quantities of plasminogen are adsorbed onto fibrin at the lysine-binding sites. Certain plasminogen activators also have a marked affinity for fibrin and are adsorbed onto it as well. The activity of the plasminogen activators may be enhanced by the presence of fibrin or fibrin monomer. Therefore, plasminogen and plasminogen activator are concentrated on the surface of the fibrin strands, where conversion of plasminogen to plasmin takes place. When the plasmin thus formed remains attached at its lysine-binding sites, it is protected from inactivation by plasmin antiplasmins. However, should the plasmin break free, exposing its lysine-binding sites, it is rapidly inactivated by alpha$_2$-antiplasmin. Any plasmin in the circulation remote from fibrin will be similarly inactivated by alpha$_2$-antiplasmin. Thus, the fibrinolytic system is a unique system in which specificity of action is determined by the ability of fibrin to adsorb both plasminogen and plasminogen activator at sites that are also involved in the inhibition of any formed plasmin. The rapidity with which free plasmin is neutralized protects other circulating proteins from plasmin digestion.[20]

CLINICAL MEASUREMENT OF FIBRINOLYSIS

The **whole blood clot lysis time** is the simplest test of fibrinolysis. If a sample of blood is allowed to clot, and that clot lyses spontaneously in 8 hours or less at 37° C, then fibrinolysis is present.

Determination of the **euglobulin lysis time** involves separation of the euglobulin fraction of plasma, which contains a portion of the plasma fibrinogen, plasminogen, and plasminogen activator. The precipitate is dissolved in buffer, clotted, then observed for clot lysis time (normal is >80 min). Factors that increase plasminogen activator levels, such as prolonged exercise, will shorten euglobulin lysis time.

Neither of the aforementioned tests distinguishes elevated plasminogen activator from elevated plasmin itself, although the latter is much less likely. Furthermore, the low levels of plasminogen activator encountered during SK or UK therapy may lead to prolonged clot lysis times. With the **fibrin plate assay**, lysis of plasminogen-free and plasminogen-containing fibrin in a Petri dish distinguishes between plasmin and plasminogen activator in the applied sample of plasma.

These tests permit a conclusion as to the current activity of the fibrinolytic system. They do not distinguish between primary and secondary fibrinolysis.

The thrombin (TT), prothrombin (PT), and partial thromboplastin (PTT) times may be prolonged during fibrinolysis owing to depletion of fibrinogen or other procoagulants. Table 4–1 summarizes laboratory findings during thrombolytic therapy with SK and UK. Current laboratory methods for determining fibrin(ogen) degradation products do not permit rapid differentiation between products from the undesirable breakdown of fibrinogen and similar products from the digestion of deposits of cross-linked fibrin.[20]

SURGERY IN THE POST-THROMBOLYTIC THERAPY PATIENT

The major concern in the patient presenting for surgery following thrombolytic therapy is hemorrhage. The clinician must contemplate the possibility of hematoma formation after insertion of lines as well as that of postoperative hemorrhage.

TABLE 4–1. CHANGES IN COMMON LABORATORY TESTS DURING THERAPY WITH SK AND UK

Test	Change	Note
Clot lysis time	↓	(or ↑ if Pg ↓↓)
Euglobulin lysis time	↓	(or ↑ if Pg ↓↓)
Lysis of Pg-fibrin plates	↑	
Plasma fibrinogen	↓	
Thrombin time	↑	Variable
Prothrombin time	↑	Variable
Partial thromboplastin time	↑	Variable

A search of the literature reveals no reports of hemorrhage from insertion of internal jugular venous or radial arterial lines following thrombolytic therapy. Perhaps this is because the number of patients undergoing surgery immediately following SK therapy has been relatively small. Although Goldberg et al. reported a SK patient who required fresh frozen plasma (FFP), platelets, cryoprecipitate (CP), and EACA to control a coagulopathy following cardiopulmonary bypass, they reported no bleeding from insertion of internal jugular venous and arterial lines even though the patient's blood was not clotting at the time of insertion.[21]

In a study of safety of SK therapy for AMI in 209 patients at six medical centers, Weinstein reports six patients with bleeding or hematoma at the puncture site, five with gastrointestinal bleeding, and two with retroperitoneal bleeding. However, five of the bleeding complications were attributable to heparin.[22]

Skinner et al. reported excessive bleeding in 17 of 24 patients undergoing coronary artery bypass grafting (CABG) within 24 hours of intravenous (IV) SK therapy. Six of these patients required administration of EACA.[23] However, other patients undergoing CABG soon after SK therapy either have not required EACA, or the treatment was not reported.[24–28]

Whether patients who have had IV SK (1 to 1.5 million units) are at greater risk for bleeding than those who have had intracoronary (IC) SK (100,000 to 300,000 units) is unclear. Cowley et al. reported an 88 per cent incidence of systemic thrombolysis in patients receiving IC SK.[29] Although Rogers noted a more profound drop in serum fibrinogen levels in patients receiving IV SK compared with those receiving IC SK, there was no difference in incidence of bleeding complications, which was low.[30]

Compared with controls, a significantly greater amount of chest tube drainage in 16 patients undergoing emergency CABG following IC SK therapy was reported by Kay et al.[31] Pilcher et al. reported that 67 per cent of 12 patients undergoing emergency CABG following SK therapy (11–IC, I–IV) required FFP, compared with 28 per cent of controls. However, there was no difference in the percentage of patients requiring re-exploration for hemorrhage.[32]

It is possible that earlier reports of hemorrhage after IV SK therapy may have been attributable to a longer duration of administration, unlike the brief, high-dose therapy currently in use.[33] From the data currently available, it would then seem that CABG within 24 hours of SK therapy is a relatively safe procedure. Although data in the literature are relatively sparse, it seems appropriate that bleeding not attributable to surgical technique should first be treated with FFP and/or CP. EACA may be reserved for those rare cases in which hemorrhage cannot be controlled with the above.

References

1. Castellino FJ: Recent advances in the fibrinolytic system. Chem Rev 81:431–446, 1981.
2. Lijnen HR, Collen D: Molecular mechanisms of thrombolytic therapy. Haemostasis 16(Suppl 3):3–15, 1986.
3. Sottrup-Jensen L, Petersen TE, Magnusson S: Human plasminogen. *In* Dayhoff MO (ed): Atlas of Protein Sequence and Structure. Vol 5, Suppl 3. Washington, DC, National Biomedical Research Foundation 1979, p 91.
4. Wallen P, Winman B: Characterization of human plasminogen. II. Separation and partial characterization of different molecular forms of human plasminogen. Biochim Biophys Acta 257:122–134, 1972.
5. Winman B, Wallen P: The specific interaction between plasminogen and fibrin. A physiological role of the lysine binding site in plasminogen. Thromb Res 10:213–222, 1977.
6. Collen D: On the regulation and control of fibrinolysis. Thromb Haemost 43:77–89, 1980.
7. Robbins KC, Summaria L, Hsieh B, et al.: The peptide chains of human plasmin. Mechanism of activation of human plasminogen to plasmin. J Biol Chem 242:2333–2342, 1967.
8. White WF, Barlow GH, Mozen MM: The isolation and characterization of plasminogen activators (urokinase) from human urine. Biochemistry 5:2160–2169, 1966.
9. Kjelgaard NO, Ploug J: Urokinase, an activator of plasminogen from human urine. II. Mechanism of plasminogen activation. Biochim Biophys Acta 24:28, 1957.
10. Paques E: Streptokinase or urokinase: The choice between them. Haemostasis 16:21–24, 1986.
11. Takada Y, Takada A: Kinetic analysis of potentiation of plasminogen activation by streptokinase in the presence of fibrin or its degradation products. Haemostasis 17:1–7, 1987.
12. Juhan-Vague I, Aillaud A, Serradimigni A: Natural inhibitors of fibrinolysis. Haemostasis 16:16–20, 1986.
13. Musumeci V: Laboratory control of urokinase therapy at low and moderate dosages. Haemostasis 13:316–321, 1983.
14. Lew AS, Ganz W: Streptokinase thrombolytic therapy in acute myocardial infarction. Haemostasis 16:113–121, 1986.
15. Collen D, Lijnen HR: Tissue-type plasminogen activator—mechanism of action and thrombolytic properties. Haemostasis 16:25–33, 1986.
16. Moroi M, Aoki N: Isolation and characterization of alpha$_2$-antiplasmin inhibitor from human plasma. J Biol Chem 251:5956–5965, 1976.
17. Bennett B, Ogston D: Role of complement, coagulation and fibrinolysis in normal haemostasis and disease. *In* Bloom AL, Thomas D (eds): Haemostasis and Thrombosis. Edinburgh, Churchill-Livingstone, 1981, pp 236–251.
18. Violand BN, Sodeta JM, Castellino FJ: The effect of epsilon aminocaproic acid on the conformation of plasminogen and plasmin. Arch Biochem Biophys 170:300–305, 1975.
19. Winman B, Collen D: Molecular mechanism of physiological fibrinolysis. Nature 272:549–550, 1978.
20. Bennett B, Ogston D: Fibrinolytic bleeding systems. *In* Ratnoff OD, Forbes CD (eds): Disorders of Hemostasis. Orlando, Grune and Stratton, 1984, pp 321–349.
21. Goldberg M, Colonna-Romano P, Babins NA: Emergency coronary artery bypass surgery following intracoronary streptokinase. Anesthesiology 61:601–604, 1984.
22. Weinstein J: Treatment of myocardial infarction with intracoronary streptokinase: Efficacy and safety data from 209 United States cases in the Hoechst-Roussel registry. Am Heart J 104:894–898, 1982.
23. Skinner JR, Phillips SJ, Zeff RH, et al.: Immediate coronary bypass following failed streptokinase infusion in evolving myocardial infarction. J Thorac Cardiovasc Surg 867:567–570, 1984.
24. Walker WE, Smalling RW, Fuentes F, et al.: Role of coronary artery bypass surgery

after intracoronary streptokinase infusion for myocardial infarction. Am Heart J 197:826–829, 1984.

25. Krebber HJ, Mathey DG, Schofer J, et al.: Indication for early aorto-coronary bypass surgery after successful intracoronary lysis. J Thorac Cardiovasc Surg 31:50–53, 1983.
26. Mathey DG, Rodeward G, Rentrop P, et al.: Intracoronary streptokinase thrombolytic recanalization and subsequent surgical bypass of remaining atherosclerotic stenosis in acute myocardial infarction: Complementary combined approach effecting reduced infarct size, preventing reinfarction, and improving left ventricular function. Am Heart J 102:1194–1201, 1981.
27. Lolley DM, Fulton R, Hamman J, et al.: Coronary artery surgery and direct coronary artery thrombolysis during acute myocardial infarction. Am Surg 49:296–300, 1983.
28. Krebber HJ, Mathey D, Kuck KJ, et al.: Management of evolving myocardial infarction by intracoronary thrombolysis and subsequent aorto-coronary bypass. J Thorac Cardiovasc Surg 83:186–193, 1982.
29. Cowley MJ, Hastillo A, Vetrovec FW, et al.: Fibrinolytic effects of intracoronary streptokinase administration in patients with acute myocardial infarction and coronary insufficiency. Circulation 67:1031–1038, 1983.
30. Rogers WJ, Mantle JA, Hood WP Jr, et al.: Prospective randomized trial of intravenous and intracoronary streptokinase in acute myocardial infarction. Circulation 68:1051–1061, 1983.
31. Kay PH, Floten S, Starr A: Emergency bypass surgery following intracoronary thrombolysis for evolving myocardial infarction. Circulation 70(Suppl 2):383, 1985.
32. Pilcher G, Morris D, Guyton R, et al.: Risk of bleeding in patients undergoing emergency coronary artery bypass graft surgery (CABG) after thrombolysis. Circulation 70(Suppl 2):384, 1985.
33. European Cooperative Study Group: Streptokinase in acute myocardial infarction. N Engl J Med 300:797–802, 1979.

CHAPTER 5

BLOOD PLASMA PRODUCTS

GLENN P. GRAVLEE and MARBRY B. HOPKINS

Over the past two decades, increased emphasis on separating whole blood into various components changed long-standing patterns of surgical blood use. Whereas whole blood served as the mainstay for many years, the need to conserve donated blood products fueled a changeover to selecting particular blood components for specific needs. While this practice soundly addressed its purpose and facilitated the care of some surgical patients, both anesthesiologists and surgeons protested the virtual elimination of whole blood availability. Our institution's principal coagulation consultant boldly proclaimed the obsolescence of whole blood at a 1982 anesthesiology didactic conference, underscoring the ineffectiveness of such protestations. As this well-motivated blood banking practice blossomed in the decade spanning 1975 to 1985, anesthesiologists and surgeons were faced with difficult decisions about appropriate indications for plasma products such as fresh frozen plasma (FFP) and cryoprecipitate (CP). Some coagulation disturbances created by extracorporeal circulation or massive transfusion apparently called for FFP, yet appropriate criteria were not scientifically established. Currently the pendulum is swinging back toward an emphasis on whole blood transfusion.[1, 2]

The use of FFP increased 10-fold in 10 years, reaching two million units in 1985.[3] A recent survey of FFP utilization in southeastern Wisconsin revealed that open-heart surgery patients utilized 42 per cent of the transfused FFP; noncardiac surgical patients utilized 26 per cent.[4] This survey of clinicians ordering FFP indicated that 61 per cent of FFP units were ordered for coagulation factors, 25 per cent for volume expansion, and 14 per cent for both reasons. Physicians considered 24 per cent of their FFP orders to be prophylactic. A chart review suggested that 32 per cent of FFP units were administered without evidence of either a coagulation disturbance or hypovolemia. Although the validity of establishing hypovolemia by chart review seems questionable, this survey demonstrates that many FFP transfusions are loosely justified at best.

In our institution, FFP was often used as a volume expander following cardiopulmonary bypass (CPB), the rationale involving replacement of depleted coagulation proteins and restoration of plasma colloid oncotic pressure to normal. Life-threatening complications arising from component therapy stimulated further thought about the appropriateness of this practice. In his memorable 1983 Rovenstine Lecture, Arthur Keats succinctly challenged such intellectual complacency in stating, "Normality is not tantamount to virtue."[5] This chapter reviews the perioperative use of three blood bank plasma products: fresh frozen plasma, single-donor plasma (SDP), and cryoprecipitate.

FRESH FROZEN PLASMA

History

In 1932, Strumia demonstrated that frozen plasma can be stored for long periods without losing any of its properties.[3] This discovery followed Rous's 1918 Nobel Prize–winning demonstration that considerable hemorrhagic hemodilution was well tolerated as long as intravascular volume was maintained. These two important discoveries combined to stimulate widespread use of frozen plasma for casualties during World War II. In the absence of immediate red blood cell (RBC) availability, this provided rapid volume expansion and temporization during cross-matching delays. In 1947, Brinkhous and colleagues demonstrated that fresh plasma corrects hemophilia in dogs.[3] The practice of freezing plasma shortly after collection to maximize preservation of labile factors soon followed their discovery. It appears that FFP was utilized sparingly in surgical patients until component therapy surged in the late 1970's.[3]

Description

To be labeled "fresh frozen plasma," plasma must be separated from whole blood and frozen within six hours of collection; it may be stored for up to one year if maintained at −18° C or lower.[6] These conditions produce minimal loss of labile clotting Factors V and VIII, which have half-lives of less than 12 hours in whole blood.[7] A typical unit contains a 200 to 250-ml volume consisting of 91 per cent water, 7 per cent protein, and 2 per cent carbohydrates and lipids. All plasma proteins remain intact, encompassing coagulation proteins, immunoglobulins, albumin, and the fibrinolytic and complement systems.

Risks and Complications

When discussing a therapeutic intervention, indications are customarily presented before complications. Owing to the aforementioned evolution of FFP clinical use, reversing that order appears appropriate. Since FFP consists of whole blood without RBC's, complications associated with its use are similar to those of whole blood. Because hemolytic transfusion reactions usually involve transfused RBC's, FFP remains exempt from hemolytic complications except for the extremely rare possibility of transfusing plasma containing abnormally high levels of antibodies against recipient RBC's. Blood banks nearly eliminate this complication by providing FFP that is ABO-compatible with the recipient, although donor antibodies outside those major groups can conceivably precipitate hemolysis. However, blood bank screening procedures eliminate major antibody carriers (including anti-D) from the FFP donor pool, rendering this possibility remote. Protein antigens present in FFP possess a limited capacity to initiate delayed antibody formation (alloimmunization) that could complicate subsequent cross-matching and transfusion.

Viral disease transmission constitutes the dominant risk in transfusing blood products. In descending order of probability, transmitted infections include non-A non-B (NANB) hepatitis, type B hepatitis, cytomegalovirus, mononucleosis, and acquired immune deficiency syndrome (AIDS).[8–10] Transmission of acute self-limited viral illnesses such as the common cold and influenza should be eliminated by donor screening procedures, but it remains possible. Similarly, bacteremia transmission is possible but unlikely. The exposure risk to viral diseases increases in proportion to the number of donors from whom the recipient receives blood products,[10] although this relationship is debatable when using volunteer blood donors exclusively.[11] It follows that products pooled from large numbers of donors, e.g., concentrates of coagulation Factors VIII and IX, produce the highest risk of transfusion-related viral diseases.[10] One unit of FFP carries the same viral transmission risk as one unit of whole blood, packed RBC's, platelets, or CP.

Hepatitis is the most common transfusion-related viral disease, occurring in 5 to 17 per cent of blood product recipients.[11–14] Of 113 transfusion-related fatalities reported to the Food and Drug Administration from 1976 through 1979, hepatitis accounted for 33.[15] Koziol and colleagues found no correlation between the transfused volume of blood products and the incidence of NANB hepatitis despite increased acquisition of anti–HBc (anti–hepatitis B core) antibody seropositivity among high volume recipients, but the small number of patients having one to five units transfused reduces the statistical power of their analysis.[14]

Accurately establishing the incidence of post-transfusion hepatitis requires scrupulous epidemiological methodology, because many cases remain subclinical. Enzyme elevations, serological markers, clinical symptoms, and jaundice peak at different times for NANB and type B hepatitis, and the incubation period and clinical course are highly variable.[10, 12, 13] Even jaundice associated with gastrointestinal (GI) symptoms can easily remain subclinical, because patients may not notice mild jaundice and often attribute GI symptoms to a flu-like syndrome. Consequently, the reported incidence of post-transfusion hepatitis can be underestimated despite fairly close follow-up. Although some might dismiss subclinical disease as insignificant, post-transfusion hepatitis derives clinical significance from potential long-term complications such as relapsing hepatitis, cirrhosis, hepatoma, and delayed progression to chronic active hepatitis.[10, 16] Since screening for hepatitis B virus has improved greatly, over 90 per cent of current post-transfusion hepatitis falls into the inadequately defined NANB category.[13] Fortunately, only 20 to 30 per cent of patients contracting NANB or type B hepatitis become jaundiced, and less than 1 per cent develop fulminant hepatitis, which is most often fatal.[10] Fulminant hepatitis is rare among NANB hepatitis patients, but many relapse during convalescence, and 10 to 50 per cent progress to chronic hepatitis.[10, 16] Donor blood now must be screened for elevated serum transaminase levels and for anti–HBc, which should reduce the prevalence of NANB virus in the donor pool by about 40 per cent. Identification of reliable NANB serological markers would prove more effective and would also exclude fewer potential donors (false-positive transaminase). Such markers have not yet been identified, so NANB hepatitis remains the most common complication of transfusion therapy.

AIDS is the delayed transfusion complication that today generates the greatest fear, justified by a two-year mortality exceeding 90 per cent once the disease is diagnosed.[17] As of June 1987, 777 cases of transfusion-related AIDS had been reported in the United States.[18] Recipients of blood products represent nearly 2 per cent of reported AIDS cases.[9] Good news for hemophiliacs is that human immunodeficiency virus (HIV, the AIDS vector) is heat-sensitive and that lyophilized concentrates of Factors VIII and IX can now be prepared using techniques that greatly reduce the possibility of AIDS transmission.[9, 19] Unfortunately, this technique can not be applied to FFP, CP, or blood without sacrificing the therapeutic efficacy of these products. Although blood products can be tested for antibody to HIV, this test can prove falsely negative in the "window" period between infection and seropositivity.[9] Although we could not find published case reports implicating FFP as the source of an AIDS infection, Conte suggests that such cases exist, and the Centers for Disease Control confirm this association.[18, 20] The risk per unit transfused (approximately 1 in 2,500 units[9]) should be identical for one unit of FFP, whole blood, packed RBC's, CP, or platelet concentrates, but the long incubation period between transfusion and symptom onset makes incidence estimates highly speculative.

Case reports link FFP with fulminant noncardiogenic pulmonary edema[21–23]; presumably this represents an anaphylactoid reaction. Although the number of reported cases remains small, personal communications indicate that many cardiovascular anesthesiologists and surgeons have suspected this FFP association in their clinical practices. To our knowledge, no prospective investigation has established the incidence of this life-threatening complication, for which treatment proves challenging. In our institution, a fatality from probable FFP-related noncardiogenic pulmonary edema caused one cardiac surgeon to eliminate routine use of FFP for postoperative volume expansion.

It is hoped that cardiogenic pulmonary edema induced by FFP fluid overload represents an infrequent complication of FFP. This complication is not unique to plasma products and can occur following excessive administration of any intravenous colloid, crystalloid, or blood product.

Indications

In 1984, the National Institutes of Health convened a multidisciplinary Consensus Development Panel, which produced a conference entitled "Fresh-Frozen Plasma: Indications and Risks."[24] Table 5–1 lists these indications, which will be discussed individually.

Isolated Factor Deficiencies. Because FFP contains all plasma proteins, it can improve deficiencies of any clotting factor. Since hemostasis requires only 10 to 40 per cent of the normal plasma concentration of the coagulation factors (I, II, V, VII, VIII, IX, X, XI, and XII),[7] replacing 15 to 20 per cent of the plasma volume (2 to 3 units or 400 to 600 ml of FFP for most adults) sufficiently replenishes plasma coagulation factor deficiencies. Large FFP volumes (600 to 2000 ml) might be needed with continuing blood losses or with clotting factor consumption from disseminated intravascular coagulation.[25] Achieving surgical hemostasis in patients having severe deficiencies of Factors VIII (classic hemophilia) or IX (hemophilia B or Christmas disease) requires replacing 30 to 40

TABLE 5–1. INDICATIONS FOR FRESH FROZEN PLASMA

1. Replacement of isolated factor deficiencies
2. Reversal of warfarin effect
3. Massive blood transfusion
4. Antithrombin-III deficiency
5. Treatment of immunodeficiencies
6. Treatment of thrombotic thrombocytopenic purpura

per cent of plasma volume. Because of the FFP volume this would require, those patients usually need pooled concentrates of the deficient factor.[3, 19] Severe fibrinogen (Factor I) deficiency may also require a more concentrated product such as CP.

Reversal of Warfarin Effect. Anticoagulation therapy with warfarin depletes the vitamin K–dependent coagulation Factors II, VII, IX, and X, as well as proteins C and S.[26, 27] Clinically significant anticoagulation from warfarin usually remits within 48 hours of the last dose (elimination half-life 37 ± 15 hours) but may last as long as five days, depending upon the commercial preparation used. Intravenous vitamin K can restore normal coagulation within six hours. In adults requiring emergency surgery, two units of FFP will neutralize warfarin's effect immediately.

Massive Blood Transfusion. Sustained blood loss replaced with only RBC transfusion clearly causes blood coagulopathies. However, since only extreme clotting factor deficiencies produce clinical bleeding, dilutional thrombocytopenia is more often implicated in coagulopathies resulting from massive blood transfusion.[28] Mannucci and colleagues prospectively investigated coagulation disturbances in 172 surgical patients requiring at least five units of whole blood and/or RBC transfusion (median: 11 units) within four hours or less.[29] Using 150,000 platelets/μl as a threshold, 85 per cent of their patients had subnormal platelet counts. Their failure to select a lower thrombocytopenia threshold (50 to 100,000/μl) to correlate with clinical bleeding undoubtedly overestimates the clinical need for platelet concentrate transfusion in their study population. Abnormalities in prothrombin time (PT) and activated partial thromboplastin time (aPTT) were found in 60 per cent and 34 per cent of their patients, respectively. Traditional criteria for disseminated intravascular coagulation were met by 30 per cent of patients. Their investigation included patient assignment to one of three groups as follows: 64 patients receiving only whole blood and/or RBC, 66 patients receiving one unit of FFP for every three units of whole blood and/or RBC, and 42 patients receiving three units of platelet concentrates and two units of FFP for every 10 units of whole blood and/or RBC. Among the three groups, the incidence of abnormalities in platelet count, fibrin(ogen) degradation products, and PT did not differ. Surprisingly, the incidence of abnormal aPTT, thrombin time (TT), and plasma fibrinogen was significantly *higher* in the prophylactic FFP group. They concluded that therapeutic intervention with FFP and platelet concentrates should be based on laboratory testing rather than on standardized therapeutic schemes.

Investigating similar patients, Counts and co-authors found that platelet counts fell in proportion to the volume of blood transfusion ($R^2 = 0.43$); whereas plasma levels of Factors V and VIII correlated poorly with transfusion volume ($R^2 = 0.15$ and 0.17, respectively), and Factor VII and fibrinogen levels were unrelated to transfusion volume.[30] Their predominant use of whole blood (750 of 893 transfused units) may explain their findings, because 59 per cent of the whole blood units they transfused were less than five days old. Whole blood preserved with citrate-phosphate-dextrose solution retains 50 per cent of Factor VIII coagulant at 24 hours and 30 per cent at 48 hours.[30, 31] This may oversimplify interpretation of Counts' study, however, because 56 per cent of their whole blood units were depleted of CP (fibrinogen and Factor VIII) before transfusion. Those investigators also found an apparent association between generalized bleeding and abnormal PT and partial thromboplastin time (PTT) values, as the mean PT (1.23 ± 0.14 times control) and PTT (1.12 ± 0.23 times control) values were higher in the patients having generalized bleeding. The specificity of these laboratory abnormalities was imperfect, however, because two of six patients having PT and PTT values ≥ 1.5 times control did not have abnormal bleeding.

The clear message from these studies is that massive transfusion produces unpredictable plasma coagulation factor abnormalities when a significant proportion of transfused RBC volume comes from whole blood. Whole blood constitutes the desired mainstay for massive transfusion, particularly if some of it has been collected within a few days of transfusion.[1, 24, 29, 30] Since transfusions even exceeding 25 units of whole blood and RBC's may not produce clinically important coagulation factor deficiencies, FFP administration should usually await documentation of significant laboratory abnormalities and clinical evidence of abnormal bleeding (e.g., oozing from surgical incision and catheter insertion sites).[32]

Defining the magnitude of laboratory abnormalities justifying FFP transfusion in the presence of bleeding proves difficult, but Table 5–2 offers some suggestions. Clinical bleeding correlates with abnormal PT, aPTT, and TT values,[29] but this association is less impressive than that observed with thrombocytopenia.[28] Even when coagulation times are

TABLE 5–2. LEVEL OF ABNORMAL COAGULATION TESTS JUSTIFYING FFP TREATMENT IF GENERALIZED BLEEDING IS PRESENT

Test	Treatment Threshold
Prothrombin time	1.3 times control*
Partial thromboplastin time	1.3 times control
Thrombin time	1.3 times control†
Fibrinogen	100 mg/dl†
Activated coagulation time	>150 seconds‡

*PT may require greater prolongation (1.5 times control) to be significant after cardiopulmonary bypass, as discussed under "Inappropriate Use of FFP"

†These abnormalities may require cryoprecipitate therapy

‡Hemochron method, another criterion being 25 seconds above the pre-operative ACT. ACT criteria based solely upon our clinical observations.

Sources: References 29, 30, 32

markedly prolonged, some patients will not experience clinical bleeding, and FFP treatment does not reliably correct the bleeding.[28, 30] Nevertheless, we believe that the abnormalities listed in Table 5–2 justify FFP if generalized bleeding is clinically evident. Because obtaining results from PT, aPTT, TT, and fibrinogen testing may require 30 to 60 minutes, the activated coagulation time (ACT) is a practical test for rapid screening (defining as abnormal Hemochron ACT values over 150 seconds). Although less sensitive than the PT, aPTT, and TT to coagulation disturbances, the ACT serves as a gross substitute for the aPTT. Simplicity and rapid availability of results in the operating suite heighten its appeal. (See Table 1–1 for a description of the ideal test of operating room coagulation.) The thromboelastogram and Sonoclot tests, can also provide helpful diagnostic information fairly quickly (see Ch. 11 and 12).

Antithrombin-III Deficiency. Antithrombin-III (AT-III) is an α_2 globulin that functions as a physiological anticoagulant.[33] Heparin binds AT-III, greatly potentiating AT-III inhibition of the coagulation cascade. Consequently, AT-III deficiency impairs heparin-induced anticoagulation.[34] Clinically important AT-III deficiencies seldom occur, but severely deficient patients occasionally present during cardiac surgery as poor responders to heparin-induced anticoagulation.[35] Despite heparin doses markedly exceeding usual requirements, ACT values may not reach levels considered safe for extracorporeal circulation (> 400 seconds).[34, 35] Causes of AT-III deficiency are discussed in Chapter 1. Mild AT-III deficiencies may influence heparin dose requirements moderately or imperceptibly, and clinically significant deficiencies respond quickly to FFP.[3, 36] AT-III also remains intact in whole blood; in the plasma it remains with RBC.[37] Although clear therapeutic guidelines have not been established, it appears advisable to administer FFP (2 to 4 units) to adult patients requiring heparin doses exceeding 700 units/kg to obtain an ACT > 400 seconds before beginning CPB.

Immunodeficiencies and Thrombotic Thrombocytopenic Purpura. FFP can be an effective treatment for infants with secondary immunodeficiency associated with protein-losing enteropathy.[24] Thrombotic thrombocytopenic purpura (TTP) is an unusual disease involving consumptive thrombocytopenia, microangiopathic hemolytic anemia, fever, and neurological and renal dysfunction. Many TTP patients improve with either FFP transfusion or plasma exchange with FFP.[38]

Inappropriate Use

Although discussed with massive transfusion, this issue should be raised again in the context of cardiac surgery requiring CPB. Current CPB practice involves hemodilution to hematocrit values between 20 and 30 per cent, which dilutes platelets and coagulation proteins pari passu with hemoglobin. Factor V levels diminish beyond those compatible with hemodilution alone,[39–42] but even Factor V levels averaging 34 per cent of normal were not associated with clinical bleeding in Mammen's study.[40] Coagulation guidelines have established 10 to 15 per cent as the minimum Factor V activity required for normal coagulation.[7] *No scientific evidence supports routine post-CPB administration of FFP to replace either coagulation proteins or the colloid oncotic activity of plasma proteins.* Most often, coagulation and other plasma proteins return to normal levels within 24 to 48 hours after CPB.[40] For volume expansion, crystalloid solutions or other colloids (5 per cent albumin or hydroxyethyl starch) are preferable to FFP.[24] Over the past 15 years, during which CPB hemodilution and anticoagulation practices have become more consistent, most investigations indicate that the dominant cause of post–CPB coagulopathy is platelet dysfunction.[39–41, 43–45] A recent review of post–CPB bleeding confirms this conclusion.[46]

Just as in massive transfusion, the use of FFP after CPB should ideally be guided by laboratory coagulation testing. Figure 5–1 suggests an algorithm for post–CPB bleeding in adult patients. Clinicians should be wary of isolated PT prolongation following CPB. Bachmann et al. found abnormal PT values in 80 per cent of patients undergoing CPB, with 36.3 per cent of patients having clinically insignificant bleeding despite PT values that should have produced coagulopathy.[47] Their investigation revealed that these patients had plasma levels of Factors II, V, VII, and X that were 70 to 80 per cent of normal, values well within the range producing normal PT values and coagulation. They postulate that a circulating inhibitor of the extrinsic coagulation system produces this misleading PT prolongation.

SINGLE DONOR PLASMA

Single donor plasma (SDP) is usually defined as plasma separated from whole blood between six hours after collection and five days after the whole blood expiration date.[6, 7] It remains stable up to five years if frozen at $-18°$ C. FFP that has been stored at $-18°$ C for over one year can be used if redesignated SDP, and recently expired thawed FFP also may meet SDP requirements. Prepared as described, SDP coagulation factor content matches FFP except for labile Factors V and VIII. The supernatant plasma remaining following CP separation also qualifies as SDP if labelled accordingly, so that clinicians will recognize its expected deficiency in fibrinogen and Factor VIII.[6] SDP adequately corrects most deficiencies of clotting factors other than Factors V, VIII, and severe Factor IX deficiency (hemophilia B). SDP should correct warfarin-induced anticoagulation as

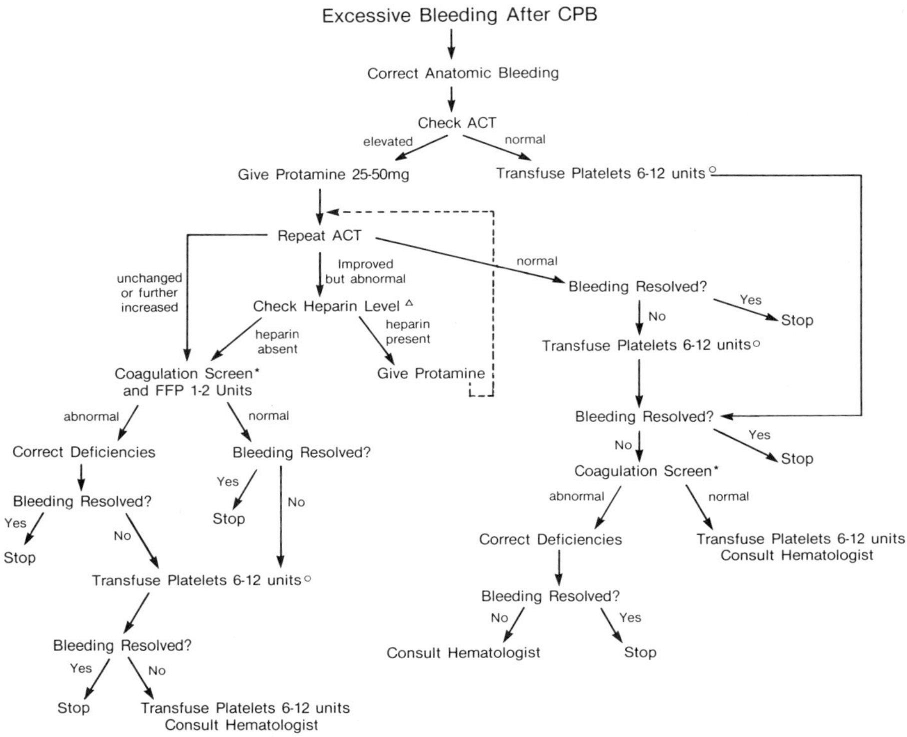

Figure 5–1. Suggested decision tree for post–CPB coagulopathy in adults.

°Some recommend deamino-8-D-arginine vasopressin (DDAVP) first, but indications are not yet clear.

ΔVarious methods can be used, most commonly in vitro protamine titration with whole blood (e.g., Hepcon) or plasma (protamine-corrected TT).

*Commonly includes PT, aPTT, TT, FDP's, and fibrinogen levels. Template bleeding time or thromboelastogram is desirable if available and technically feasible.

proficiently as FFP does. Similarly, SDP fully corrects deficiencies of antithrombin III and immune globulins.[3, 48]

Does SDP have an advantage over FFP? SDP costs slightly less than FFP, carries the same complications and risks, and represents a valid blood bank plasma conservation technique, especially in salvaging plasma from outdated whole blood. However, SDP has not gained widespread acceptance.[48]

CRYOPRECIPITATE

History

When blood was first stored at 0 to 6° C early in this century, the formation of a plasma precipitate was soon recognized. In 1965, Pool determined that the content of this precipitate could have therapeutic value, described a method for isolating it from FFP, and may have affixed the prefix "cryo" (cold) to this product.[19] CP availability produced a major advance in the treatment of classic hemophilia and von Willebrand's disease.

Description

CP forms from FFP thawed at 4° C, after which all but 10 to 15 ml of the supernatant plasma is removed. CP can be stored at −18° C for 12 months, and it contains a concentrated solution of Factor VIII:C (procoagulant), Factor VIII:vWF (von Willebrand's factor), fibrinogen, Factor XIII, and fibronectin.[7] Each unit (bag) contains approximately half the amount of the Factor VIII, 20 to 30 per cent of the Factor XIII, and 20 to 40 per cent of the fibrinogen (150 to 250 mg) present in one FFP unit, in 2 to 4 per cent of the volume.

Risks and Complications

Therapeutic efficacy usually mandates pooling 10 or more units of CP, and the transmission risk for blood-borne viral disease correlates with the size of the donor pool to which the recipient is exposed. Therefore, the use of 10 to 20 units of CP increases the chance of disease transmission. Hemophiliacs have acquired AIDS from CP.[2, 9] CP contains anti-A and anti-B alloagglutinins, so large transfusions of ABO-incompatible CP can generate hemolysis, hence ABO-compatibility is recommended but not required. Overtransfusion with CP can produce elevated fibrinogen levels and increase the risk of intravascular thrombosis.[7]

Indications

CP is indicated in the treatment of hemophilia A, von Willebrand's disease types II and III, and deficiencies of Factor XIII or fibrinogen. Classic type I von Willebrand's disease responds to the synthetic agent deamino-8-D-arginine vasopression (DDAVP, see Ch. 9).[19] Patients undergoing liver transplantation may require CP transfusions to replace severely depleted fibrinogen and Factor VIII. In many situations, consultation with a hematologist specializing in coagulation appears advisable before transfusing CP, because other therapies may be preferred, and the appropriate number of CP units may be difficult to determine.

Both CP and FFP have been used in small volumes as components of topical glue during cardiothoracic procedures.[49–51] This practice might place patients at risk for blood-borne disease transmission, so it may be preferable to utilize bovine topical thrombin for this purpose.

Use After Cardiopulmonary Bypass

Having prospectively observed a high incidence of fibrinolysis, Lambert, Marengo-Rowe, and co-authors recommended using CP in bleeding post–CPB patients not responding to empirical therapy with epsilon-aminocaproic acid (EACA).[52] In this 1979 study, 164 of 774 patients received EACA "with or without cryoprecipitate or fresh-frozen plasma." Recently, Marengo-Rowe reaffirmed these recommendations,[53] suggesting CP utilization after observing a low plasma fibrinogen concentration (defined in the 1979 study as < 225 mg/dl[52]) when EACA therapy fails to arrest post–CPB bleeding (see Ch. 4). This group's findings contrast sharply with those of other studies of post–CPB bleeding, particularly in their virtual dismissal of platelet dysfunction as an important etiology.[39–41, 43–45] Bick points out that while many have identified fibrinolytic activity during and after CPB, controlled studies have not demonstrated any advantage to routine use of EACA; thus he believes that EACA is rarely needed.[46] In a prospective evaluation of 466 cardiac surgical patients conducted at our institution, 15.7 per cent of patients developed post–CPB fibrin(ogen) degradation product (FDP) titers exceeding 32 μg/ml, and these levels correlated with clinical postoperative blood loss ($p < 0.05$).[54] However, 5 of 18 patients having FDP titers exceeding 64 μg/ml did not bleed excessively. In all cases, hemostasis was achieved without using CP, and EACA was administered to only 9 patients. On the basis of these data, and in view of risks of disease transmission, the use of EACA, FFP, and CP as recommended by Lambert et al. and Marengo-Rowe would seem to be unduly liberal.[52, 53]

"SHOTGUN" THERAPY

Sometimes overwhelming blood loss makes it difficult or impossible to await laboratory results before initiating transfusions directed specifically at coagulopathy correction. Assuming complete post–CPB heparin neutralization, massive transfusion and post–CPB coagulopathies more often call for platelet concentrates (or possibly DDAVP) than for FFP. Because fresh whole blood is usually unavailable, empirical use of FFP after CPB in infants seems reasonable if protamine fails to normalize the ACT. Although FFP use cannot be strictly limited to laboratory-documented plasma coagulation factor deficiencies, it appears that many clinicians could accomplish this more often than they do.[3, 4] We see no reason to transfuse CP without laboratory tests documenting its need. Blood banks are increasing surveillance of transfusion practices in a salutary effort to reduce inappropriate transfusions.[1]

Amidst the hectic activity surrounding unstable surgical patients who appear also to have a coagulopathy, it becomes all too easy to seek quick solutions while paying insufficient attention to long-term transfusion hazards. Even a small risk becomes significant when the benefit derived is questionable. If physicians will recognize these dangers they will transfuse blood bank products, while exercising the same care utilized by anesthesiologists in selecting anesthetic techniques and by surgeons in selecting operative approaches. If "shotgun" therapy of a coagulopathy becomes essential, we advise firing one barrel at a time. In most clinical situations, current knowledge suggests that empirical platelet concentrate transfusion should precede empirical FFP transfusion.

References

1. Grindon AJ, Tomasulo PS, Bergin JJ, et al.: The hospital transfusion committee: Guidelines for improving practice. JAMA 253:540–543, 1985.
2. Widmann FK (ed): Adverse effects of blood transfusion. *In* Technical Manual. Arlington, VA, American Association of Blood Banks, 1985, pp 325–344.
3. Oberman HA: Uses and abuses of fresh frozen plasma. *In* Garratty G (ed): Current Concepts in Transfusion Therapy. Arlington, VA, American Association of Blood Banks, 1985, pp 110–124.
4. Snyder AJ, Gottschall JL, Menitove JE: Why is fresh-frozen plasma transfused? Transfusion 26:107–112, 1986.
5. Keats AS: The Rovenstine Lecture, 1983: Cardiovascular anesthesia: Perceptions and perspectives. Anesthesiology 60:467–474, 1984.
6. Widmann FK (ed): Blood and blood components: Preparation, storage and shipment. *In* Technical Manual. Arlington, VA, American Association of Blood Banks, 1985, pp 35–58.
7. Snyder EL (ed): Blood Transfusion Therapy: A Physician's Handbook. Arlington, VA, American Association of Blood Banks, 1983, pp 19–27.
8. Drew WL, Miner RC: Transfusion-related cytomegalovirus infection following noncardiac surgery. JAMA 247:2389–2391, 1982.
9. Kunkel SE, Warner MA: Human T-cell lymphotropic virus type III (HTLV-III) infection: How it can affect you, your patients, and your anesthesia practice. Anesthesiology 66:195–207, 1987.
10. Widmann FK (ed): Hepatitis. *In* Technical Manual. Arlington, VA, American Association of Blood Banks, 1985, pp 345–358.
11. Aach RD, Kahn RA: Post-transfusion hepatitis: Current perspectives. Ann Intern Med 92:539–546, 1980.
12. Editorial: Post-transfusion-hepatitis. Br Med J 283:1–2, 1981.
13. Editorial: Non-A, non-B hepatitis. Lancet 2:1077–1078, 1984.
14. Koziol DE, Holland PV, Alling DW, et al.: Antibody to hepatitis B core antigen as a paradoxical marker for non-A, non-B hepatitis agents in donated blood. Ann Intern Med 104:488–495, 1986.
15. Myhre BA: Fatalities from blood transfusion. JAMA 244:1333–1335, 1980.
16. Hornbrook MC, Dodd RY, Jacobs P, et al.: Reducing the incidence of non-A, non-B post-transfusion hepatitis by testing donor blood for alanine aminotransferase. N Engl J Med 307:1315–1321, 1982.
17. Hardy AM, Rauch K, Echenberg D, et al.: The economic impact of the first 10,000 cases of acquired immunodeficiency syndrome in the United States. JAMA 255:209–211, 1986.
18. Drotman P: Personal communication Centers for Disease Control, Atlanta, Georgia, 1987.

19. Lusher JM: Replacement therapy for congenital and acquired disorders of blood coagulation: Available products. *In* Garratty G (ed): Current Concepts in Transfusion Therapy. Arlington, VA, American Association of Blood Banks, 1985, pp 27–49.
20. Conte JE: Infection with human immunodeficiency virus in the hospital: Epidemiology, infection control, and biosafety considerations. Ann Intern Med 105:730–736, 1986.
21. O'Connor PC, Erskine JG, Pringle TH: Pulmonary oedema after transfusion with fresh frozen plasma. Br Med J 282:379–380, 1981.
22. Culliford AT, Thomas S, Spencer FC: Fulminating noncardiogenic pulmonary edema: A newly recognized hazard during cardiac operations. J Thorac Cardiovasc Surg 80:868–875, 1980.
23. Hashim SW, Kay HR, Hammond GL, et al.: Noncardiogenic pulmonary edema after cardiopulmonary bypass: An anaphylactic reaction to fresh frozen plasma. Am J Surg 147:560–564, 1984.
24. Tullis JL, Alving B, Bove JR, et al.: Fresh-frozen plasma: Indications and risks. JAMA 253:551–553, 1985.
25. Brauenstein AH, Oberman HA: Transfusion of plasma components. Transfusion 24:281–286, 1984.
26. Ellison N, Jobes DR, Schwartz AJ: Implications of anticoagulant therapy. *In* Stehling LC (ed): Techniques of Blood Transfusion. Int Anesthesiol Clin 20:121–135, 1982.
27. O'Reilly RA: Anticoagulant, antithrombotic, and thrombolytic drugs. *In* Gilman AG, Goodman LS, Rall TW, Murad F (eds): Goodman and Gilman's The Pharmacological Basis of Therapeutics (ed 7). New York, MacMillan, 1985, pp 1338–1359.
28. Miller RD, Robbins TO, Tong MJ, Barton SL: Coagulation defects associated with massive blood transfusions. Ann Surg 174:794–801, 1976.
29. Mannucci PM, Federici AB, Sirchia G: Hemostasis testing during massive blood replacement: A study of 172 cases. Vox Sang 41:113–123, 1982.
30. Counts RB, Haisch C, Simon TL, et al.: Hemostasis in massively transfused trauma patients. Ann Surg 190:91–99, 1979.
31. Nilsson L, Hedner U, Nilsson IM, Robertson B: Shelf-life of bank blood and stored plasma with special reference to coagulation factors. Transfusion 23:377–381, 1983.
32. White GC, Marder VJ, Colman RW, et al.: Approach to the bleeding patient. *In* Colman RW, Hirsh J, Marder VJ, and Salzman EW (eds): Hemostasis and Thrombosis (ed 2). Philadelphia, JB Lippincott Company, 1987, pp 1048–1060.
33. Cosgriff TM, Bishop DT, Hershgold MH, et al.: Familial antithrombin III deficiency: Its natural history, genetics, diagnosis and treatment. Medicine 62:209–220, 1983.
34. Esposito RA, Culliford AT, Colvin SB, et al.: Heparin resistance during cardiopulmonary bypass: The role of heparin pretreatment. J Thorac Cardiovasc Surg 85:346–353, 1983.
35. Mabry CD, Read RC, Thompson BW, et al.: Identification of heparin resistance during cardiac and vascular surgery. Arch Surg 114:129–134, 1979.
36. Sabbagh AH, Chung GKT, Shuttleworth P, et al.: Fresh frozen plasma: A solution to heparin resistance during cardiopulmonary bypass. Ann Thorac Surg 37:466–468, 1984.
37. Lundsgaard-Hansen P, Ehrengruber E, Frei E, et al.: Antithrombin III and related parameters in surgical patients receiving blood components. Vox Sang 46:19–28, 1983.
38. Eisenstaedt RS, Colman RW, Marder VJ: Thrombotic thrombocytopenic purpura. *In* Colman RW, Hirsh J, Marder VJ, and Salzman EW (eds): Hemostasis and Thrombosis (ed 2). Philadelphia, JB Lippincott Company, 1987, pp 1016–1025.
39. Kalter RD, Saul CM, Wetstein L, et al.: Cardiopulmonary bypass: Associated hemostatic abnormalities. J Thorac Cardiovasc Surg 77:427–435, 1979.
40. Mammen EF, Koets MH, Washington BC, et al.: Hemostasis changes during cardiopulmonary bypass surgery. Semin Thromb Hemost 11:281–292, 1985.
41. Moriau M, Masure R, Hurlet A, et al.: Haemostasis disorders in open heart surgery with extracorporeal circulation: Importance of the platelet function and the heparin neutralization. Vox Sang 32:41–51, 1977.
42. Müller S, Popov-Cenič S, Büttner W, et al.: Studies of fibrinolytic and coagulation of factors during open heart surgery. II. Postoperative bleeding tendency and changes in the coagulation system. Thromb Res 7:589–598, 1975.

43. Friedenberg WR, Myers WO, Plotka ED, et al.: Platelet dysfunction associated with cardiopulmonary bypass. Ann Thorac Surg 25:298–305, 1978.
44. Harker LA, Malpass TW, Branson HE, et al.: Mechanism of abnormal bleeding in patients undergoing cardiopulmonary bypass: Acquired transient platelet dysfunction associated with selective α-granule release. Blood 56:824–834, 1980.
45. McKenna R, Bachmann F, Whittaker B, et al.: The hemostatic mechanism after open-heart surgery. II. Frequency of abnormal platelet functions during and after extracorporeal circulation. J Thorac Cardiovasc Surg 70:298–308, 1975.
46. Bick RL: Hemostasis defects associated with cardiac surgery, prosthetic devices, and other extracorporeal circuits. Semin Thromb Hemost 11:249–280, 1985.
47. Bachmann F, McKenna R, Cole ER, Najafi H: The hemostatic mechanism after open-heart surgery. I. Studies on plasma coagulation factors and fibrinolysis in 512 patients after extracorporeal circulation. J Thorac Cardiovasc Surg 70:76–85, 1975.
48. Oberman HA: Inappropriate use of fresh-frozen plasma (editorial). JAMA 253:556–557, 1985.
49. Dresdale A, Bowman FO Jr, Malm JR, et al.: Hemostatic effectiveness of fibrin glue derived from single-donor fresh frozen plasma. Ann Thorac Surg 40:385–387, 1985.
50. Lupinetti FM, Stoney WS, Alford WC Jr, et al.: Cryoprecipitate-topical thrombin glue: Initial experience in patients undergoing cardiac operations. J Thorac Cardiovasc Surg 90:502–505, 1985.
51. Robicsek F, Born GVR: The control of bleeding after cardiopulmonary bypass by the intrapericardial instillation of fresh frozen plasma and platelets with microfibrillar collagen. Thorac Cardiovasc Surg 32:127–130, 1984.
52. Lambert CJ, Marengo-Rowe AJ, Leveson JE, et al.: The treatment of postperfusion bleeding using ϵ-aminocaproic acid, cryoprecipitate, fresh-frozen plasma, and protamine sulfate. Ann Thorac Surg 28:440–444, 1979.
53. Marengo-Rowe AJ: The experts opine. Surv Anesth 30:377–379, 1986.
54. Stuart JJ, Cordell AR, Gravlee GP, Lavender SW: Mechanisms of hemorrhage in patients undergoing cardiopulmonary bypass surgery (abstract). Thromb Haemost 54:157, 1985.

CHAPTER 6

PLATELET FUNCTION ALTERATIONS DURING CARDIAC SURGERY*

FREDERICK W. CAMPBELL
and V. PAUL ADDONIZIO, Jr.

> . . . Abnormal bleeding after cardiopulmonary bypass is usually not due to 1) a reduction in the levels and function of coagulation factors, 2) heparinization or the possibility of subsequent inadequate neutralization or protamine excess, 3) qualitative defects in the polymerization of fibrin, or 4) increased fibrinolytic activity and the secondary effect of fibrin-fibrinogen degradation products on coagulation. By contrast, available data persuasively demonstrate that postbypass hemorrhage is most often due to an acute acquired defect in the formation of the platelet plug.
>
> *Laurence Harker*[1]

Despite the success of open-heart surgery, postoperative bleeding is a persistent cause for concern because it results in hemorrhagic complications and requires re-exploration of the chest in 3 per cent of patients who undergo cardiac operations.[1a] While many hemostatic defects may be observed in patients following cardiopulmonary bypass (CPB), the most predictable defect resulting from open-heart surgery is platelet dysfunction.

Although quantitative and qualitative platelet deficiencies are produced by a variety of factors occurring in the perioperative period (Table 6–1), extracorporeal circulation is clearly the major source of the iatrogenic platelet disturbance. Unfortunately, the mechanisms of platelet injury during extracorporeal circulation may be poorly understood by

*This work was supported in part by funds from the National Institutes of Health Grant HL 34026.

TABLE 6–1. FACTORS IN CARDIAC SURGERY RESPONSIBLE FOR QUANTITATIVE AND QUALITATIVE PLATELET DEFICIENCIES AND POSSIBLE MECHANISMS OF ANTIPLATELET ACTION

	Quantitative Deficiencies (Thrombocytopenia)	Qualitative Deficiencies (Platelet Dysfunction)
Cardiopulmonary bypass		
Hemodilution		—
Membrane oxygenators	a	a
Bubble oxygenators	x,a	x,a
Cardiotomy suction	x,a	x,a
Filters	x,a	x,a
Hypothermia	s	i
Drugs		
Preoperative platelet inhibitor therapy	—	i
Heparin	s,a?	a?
Protamine	s,a?	a?
Blood transfusion	d	a?
Cardiovascular adjuvant drugs	—	i
Anesthetic agents	—	i
Others		
Pulmonary artery catheters	x?,a?	—

Mechanisms (see text)
a = Platelet activation
d = Dilution of circulating platelets
i = Direct inhibition of platelet cellular function
s = Transient sequestration of platelets
x = Mechanical platelet injury or destruction

the clinicians who conduct CPB and who must treat possible postoperative bleeding. Understanding platelet function and the perioperative factors that impair platelet function should allow the anesthesiologist and surgeon to recognize those instances in which postoperative hemorrhage is due to platelet deficiencies and to suggest appropriate therapeutic strategies.

PLATELET ANATOMY

Prior to consideration of platelet behavior during extracorporeal circulation, it is appropriate to review current concepts of platelet structure and function. The reader is referred to texts[2, 3] and reviews[4] for detailed descriptions of platelet anatomy and function. Four functional anatomical zones may be identified in the platelet cell (Fig. 6–1). Each is related to specific aspects of platelet function.

Cell Membrane

The cell membrane consists of a trilaminar phospholipid plasma membrane and an exterior glycoprotein coat. Functionally, the cell

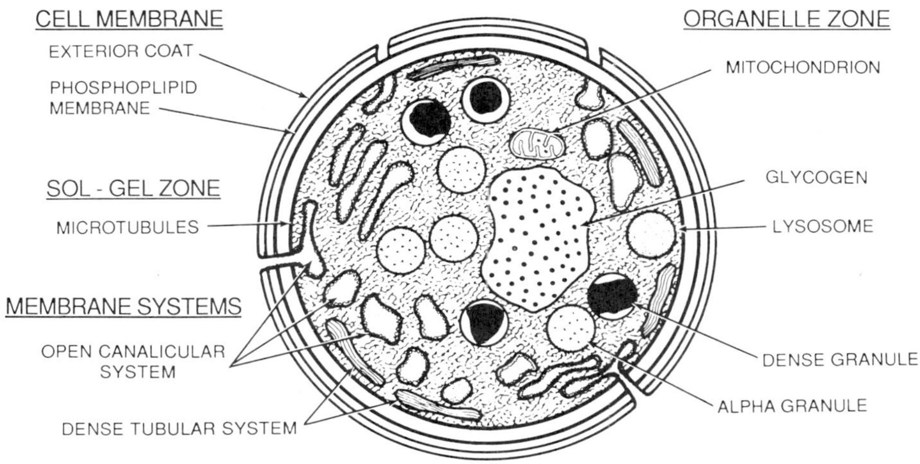

Figure 6–1. Anatomy of the platelet cell is depicted in this horizontal section. Four groups of cell structures may be distinguished on the basis of their roles in platelet function and their intracellular location.

At the cell perimeter, the phospholipid **cell membrane** contains receptors providing mechanisms by which extracellular physical and chemical agents may activate intracellular processes. The glycoprotein coat on the cell surface permits platelet adhesion and aggregation.

The **sol-gel zone** in the peripheral cytoplasm is the location of circumferentially arranged microtubules responsible for the discoid shape of the normal platelet. Contractile elements within the microtubules induce a functional shape change in the activated platelet.

The **organelle zone** in the central cytoplasm contains alpha, dense, and lysosome granules. The granule contents are actively secreted from the stimulated platelet to promote the hemostatic process. Mitochondria and glycogen particles are also located in this intracellular zone.

Intracellular membranes are situated in the platelet cytoplasm. **The open canalicular system** located throughout the cytoplasm connects the cell interior with the surface, thereby increasing the cell surface area and facilitating the secretion of platelet granules. The **dense tubular system** lies in the peripheral cytoplasm close to the sol-gel zone. It is a reservoir of platelet calcium and the site of arachidonate metabolism and thromboxane A_2 synthesis.

membrane provides (1) physical sites for adhesion to endothelial surfaces and aggregation with other platelets, (2) platelet factor 3 (lipid coagulation activator, (3) receptors for agonists (e.g., collagen, ADP, thrombin, fibrinogen, thromboxane A_2) which stimulate platelet activation, and (4) a coupling mechanism for transferring the triggering stimulus from the platelet surface to the platelet interior where the activation process occurs.

Sol-Gel Zone

In the peripheral cytoplasm of the platelet is located a circumferential arrangement of microtubules and actin- and myosin-containing microfilaments. These are responsible for maintaining the normal discoid shape of the unstimulated platelet. Early in the platelet activation process, calcium-mediated actin-catalyzed contraction of the myosin components of the microfilaments transforms the disc-shaped platelet into a sphere, extrudes pseudopods, and centralizes the platelet secretory granules.

Organelle Zone

The central cytoplasm of the platelet contains at least three types of platelet secretory granules as well as mitochondria and glycogen particles. The contents of the alpha, dense, and lysosome granules and their biological activities[5, 6] are listed in Table 6–2. When platelet activation proceeds sufficiently, the contents of the secretory granules are actively extruded from the platelet. The secretion process, commonly termed the

TABLE 6–2. CONTENTS OF PLATELET SECRETORY GRANULES AND THEIR PHYSIOLOGICAL ACTIVITIES

Secretory Granules and Contents	Physiological Activities
1. Alpha granules	
Coagulation factors	Co-factors for enzymatic coagulation cascade
Fibrinogen	
Factor V	
Platelet-specific proteins	PF4 potentiates ADP-induced platelet aggregation and has antiheparin activity
Platelet factor 4 (PF4)	
Low affinity platelet factor 4 (B thromboglobulin)	LA-PF4 possesses antiheparin activity
Cationic proteins	
Mitogenic factor	Stimulates vascular smooth muscle growth
Permeability factor	Increases endothelial permeability
Chemotactic factor	Attracts leukocytes
Bactericidal factor	Promotes mild antimicrobial activity
Glycoproteins	Participate in cell adhesion and cell-to-cell interactions
2. Dense granules	
Adenine nucleotides (ADP, ATP)	ADP stimulates platelet aggregation and secretion
Guanosine nucleotides (GDP, GTP)	Function unknown
Pyrophosphate	No physiological function
Calcium	Uncertain, promotes coagulation
Serotonin	Vasoconstriction, stimulates platelet aggregation and secretion in non-human species
3. Lysosomes	
Acid hydrolases	May exert hydrolytic activity in acid environments
Neutral proteases	May propagate vascular damage and promote vascular permeability

"release reaction," occurs by exocytosis and requires cellular ATP, intracellular calcium, and platelet microfilament contraction. There is a dose-response relationship between the platelet-activing stimulus and the extent of the resulting activation process. Relatively weak agonists (ADP, epinephrine, synthetic surfaces) result in the secretion of alpha and dense granules. The chemical mediators released from these granules contribute to hemostasis by triggering the recruitment and activation of other platelets, accelerating the coagulation cascade, and inducing local vasoconstriction and increased vascular permeability. Stronger agonists such as thrombin and collagen induce the secretion of lysosomes as well as alpha and dense granules from the platelet.

Membrane Systems

The surface connecting open canalicular system is a series of tortuous invaginations of the cell membrane found distributed throughout the platelet cytoplasm which functionally increase the cell surface area exponentially. The open canalicular system increases the number of membrane receptor sites, brings the agonist-receptor interaction into the cell interior close to the intracellular sites of the activation process, and facilitates the extrusion of secreted platelet granule contents to the exterior.

Structurally, the dense tubular system is closely related to the open canalicular system and the circumferential microtubules of the sol-gel zone. This membrane system performs two vital roles. The dense tubular system is the intracellular calcium reservoir, analogous to the sarcotubules in muscle fibers. Calcium is an important mediator of a number of platelet functions, including microfilament contraction, granule secretion, and arachidonic acid metabolism. The dense tubular system is also the intracellular site of the enzymes involved in arachidonic acid metabolism and prostaglandin synthesis. Upon platelet activation, calcium-mediated phospholipases generate arachidonic acid from platelet phospholipids. Arachidonic acid is then converted by the enzyme cyclooxygenase to cyclic endoperoxides (prostaglandins G_2 [PGG_2] and H_2 [PGH_2] and thromboxane A_2 (Fig. 6–2). The production of thromboxane A_2 serves to catalyze the hemostatic process by mediating the subsequent secretion of platelet granule contents, triggering activation of other circulating platelets, and inducing local vasoconstriction.

PLATELET FUNCTION

Platelet Activation

Platelet activation contributes to normal hemostasis by (1) causing platelet adhesion to disrupted vascular endothelial surfaces, (2) triggering

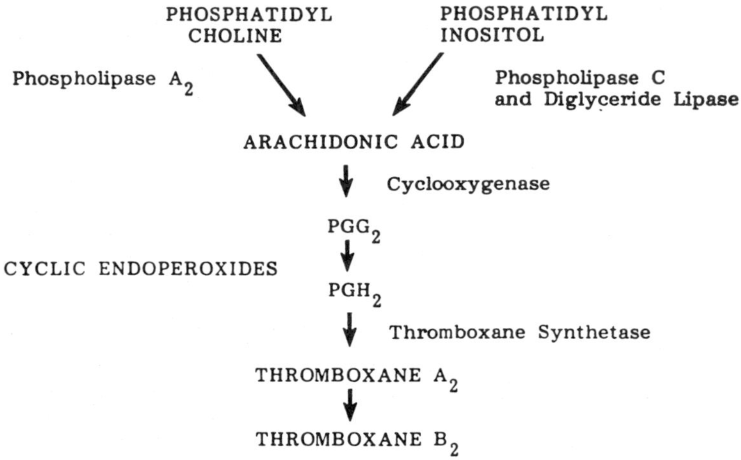

Figure 6–2. Schematic representation of the pathway of thromboxane A_2 synthesis in the platelet. Platelet membrane phospholipids are converted to arachidonic acid by phospholipases in the stimulated platelet. Arachidonic acid is cyclo-oxygenated to form prostaglandin G_2 (PGG_2), which rapidly undergoes peroxidation to prostaglandin H_2 (PGH_2). The conversion of arachidonate to PGG_2 is catalyzed by the enzyme cyclo-oxygenase. Platelet inhibitors such as aspirin and nonsteroidal anti-inflammatory agents inhibit cyclo-oxygenase activity.

In the platelet, the enzyme thromboxane synthetase catalyzes the conversion of PGH_2 to thromboxane A_2. This substance is one of the most potent platelet agonists known and is a powerful vasoconstrictor. Once released from the platelet, thromboxane is unstable in plasma and is rapidly hydrated to the stable, but inactive, thromboxane B_2.

platelet-to-platelet adhesion (aggregation) resulting in the formation of the platelet plug, (3) contributing co-factors (platelet factor 3, alpha and dense granule products) to the enzymatic coagulation cascade generating fibrin strand formation, and (4) inducing local vasoconstriction. Platelet activation is normally triggered by ADP or collagen in exposed endothelial basement membranes and perivascular tissue, by thrombin and fibrinogen from blood, and by thromboxane A_2, ADP, and fibrinogen secreted from other platelets. It occurs at a rate and to an extent determined by the nature and concentration of the stimulating factors, as well as by the sensitivity of the circulating platelets.

Teleologically, the graded response of platelets to agonists triggering their activation is protective in nature. If platelet reaction were an "all or none" phenomenon, complete intravascular coagulation could occur as a result of a minor stimulus. This graded response develops with a series of sequential intracellular functions (Fig. 6–3). The stronger the inciting trigger, the further along this sequence the activation process proceeds. The resulting platelet behavior may be observed in vitro by

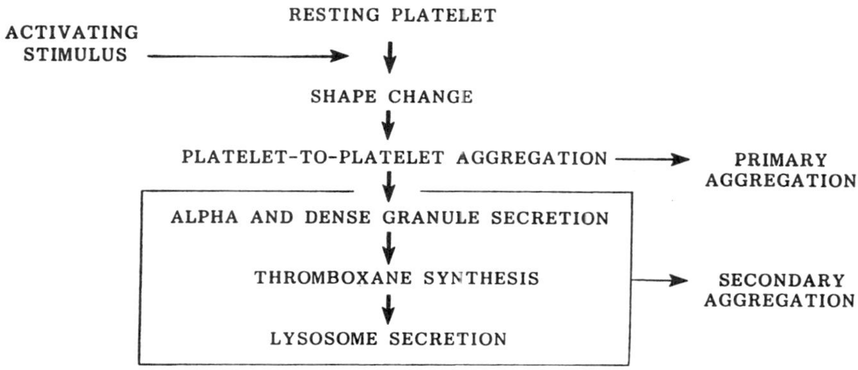

Figure 6–3. A schematic representation of the basic platelet activation response. An activating stimulus triggers a sequence of steps resulting in platelet function. The strength of the inciting stimulus and the sensitivity of the platelet will determine how far along this sequence the activation process proceeds. Weak stimuli and dysfunctional platelets may result in shape change or platelet-to-platelet adhesion only. Platelet-to-platelet adhesion causes primary platelet aggregation. Without further stimulation, the activation sequence may stop and be reversed. The platelets will disaggregate and be restored to a normal discoid shape.

Increasing concentrations of stimulating agonists exposed to healthy platelets will trigger alpha and dense granule release and thromboxane A_2 synthesis. A very potent stimulus is required to induce lysosome acid hydrolase secretion. The phase of granule secretion and thromboxane synthesis is termed the **release reaction** and is an irreversible process committing the platelet to degranulation. The platelet secretory products released cause secondary platelet aggregation, formation in the in vivo platelet plug, activation of the enzymatic coagulation cascade, and localized vascular changes.

means of platelet aggregometry (Fig. 6–4). The initial steps in the activation sequence are induced by stimuli that are weak in nature or low in concentration. The first observable response in the activation sequence is a change in platelet shape from discoid to spherical and results from microfilament contraction. Without further platelet stimulation, the normal discoid shape is restored. Primary aggregation occurs with increasing concentrations or more potent agonists. A change in the exterior glycoprotein coat of the platelet cell membrane occurs together with the change in platelet shape and creates a sticky cell surface, resulting in platelet-to-platelet adhesion and primary aggregation. Primary aggregation is partial in degree and, without the addition of further stimuli, reverses gradually. The platelets separate and restore their normal appearance. To this point, the activation sequence is reversible and does not compromise platelet function. With increasing doses of platelet agonists, secondary platelet aggregation occurs. Secondary aggregation is associated with prostaglandin synthesis and granule secretion and is irreversible. Dense and alpha granules are released earlier in the secondary aggregation phase, while lysosomes are released later. Further

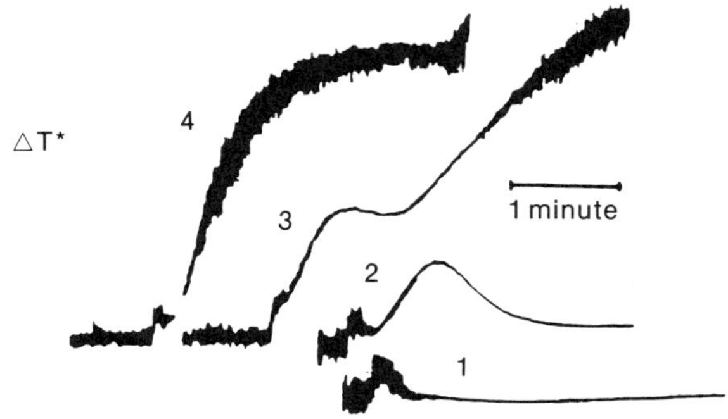

* △T—change in light transmission

Figure 6–4. The graded response of platelets to increasing concentrations of a platelet agonist is depicted in four in vitro aggregation curves. The curves were obtained by combining turbid platelet-rich plasma (PRP) with increasing amounts of an agonist (thrombin) in a platelet aggregometer.

The platelet aggregometer measures the extent of platelet aggregation, an observable manifestation of platelet activation. This photo-optical instrument measures light transmittance through samples of platelet-containing plasma. PRP is normally turbid and transmits light poorly. When activating agonists are added, stimulating platelet activation and causing aggregation, the turbidity of the plasma decreases. Light transmittance through the plasma sample progressively increases with the formation of increasingly large platelet aggregates. The amount of light transmitted is then recorded and produces an aggregation curve. With increasing degrees of platelet aggregation, the reduction in turbidity and change in light transmittance are greater, and the corresponding curves show larger upward deflections from the baseline.

In curve 1, PRP is combined with thrombin 0.05 units/ml. Platelet shape change indicated by narrowing of the baseline took place within a few seconds, but aggregation did not occur. Within 10 min, the baseline recovers its normal amplitude as platelet discoid shape is restored (not shown).

In curve 2, where PRP is combined with thrombin 0.1 unit/ml, upward deflection of the tracing indicates that a change in light transmittance occurred after shape change had developed. The change in light transmission coincides with an initial wave of primary aggregation. Platelet clumps dispersed completely in this sample as indicated by a decrease in light transmittance and a return of the recording to baseline. Platelet discoid shape is restored and the baseline recovers its normal amplitude within 10 min (not shown).

Curve 3, recorded when PRP was exposed to thrombin 0.15 unit/ml, demonstrates that an initial phase of primary aggregation was followed by a brief period in which disaggregation began. This pause was followed by a rapid increase in light transmission as a second wave of aggregation took place. This secondary aggregation is entirely dependent for its initiation on endogenous products extruded from platelets during the "release reaction."

Curve 4 was obtained when PRP was treated with thrombin 0.18 unit/ml. The first and second waves of aggregation are fused together, obscuring the biphasic nature of the platelet response. This occurred because the high concentration of agonist caused acceleration of the platelet activation sequence and rapid development of secondary aggregation. (Modified from White JG: Platelet morphology and function. *In* Williams WJ, Beutler E, Erslev AJ, Lichtman MA (eds): Hematology (ed 3). New York, McGraw-Hill, 1983.)

increases in the dose or potency of inciting agonists accelerate the rate of secondary aggregation.

Intracellular Regulation of Platelet Function

Physiological triggering of platelet activation occurs as specific agonists from sources outside the cell bind to specific receptors on the external platelet cell membrane. In order for the platelet activation process to be initiated, a stimulus-response coupling mechanism must transfer the triggering stimulus from the surface receptors to the platelet cytoplasm where the activation process takes place. The pathways through which the stimulus-response coupling occurs serve as means for possible intracellular regulation of platelet activity. The precise nature of the platelet's regulatory and coupling mechanisms is not known with certainty. It is clear, however, that at least three coupling pathways exist: an ADP-dependent pathway, a platelet-activating factor (PAF, or PAF-acether) pathway, and an arachidonic acid pathway.[7] The specific nature of the triggeriing agonist, through its receptor, determines which pathway(s) is (are) of importance in initiating the platelet activation sequence.

Thromboxane A_2 is generated from arachidonic acid in the stimulated platelet. In addition to its role as a recruiter and activator of other platelets when released from the cell, thromboxane A_2 promotes the intracellular platelet activation sequence. The mechanisms by which thromboxane A_2, as well as the cyclic endoperoxides, exert these intracellular actions are not known. Nevertheless, many drugs inhibit platelet activation and function by inhibiting cyclo-oxygenase and the production of thromboxane A_2 (see Fig. 6–2), thus interrupting this coupling pathway. Examples include aspirin, indomethacin, and nonsteroidal anti-inflammatory agents.

While it is clear that thromboxane A_2 and cyclic endoperoxides are potent mediators of platelet aggregation and secretion, there is evidence that they are not essential mediators of these events.[8, 9] For example, platelets react vigorously to thrombin or collagen, despite inhibition of cyclo-oxygenase by aspirin, indomethacin, or other nonsteroidal anti-inflammatory agents.[10]

Associated with the pathways of stimulus-response coupling are important intracellular mediators that modulate the triggering, coupling, and activation processes. Cyclic AMP and intracellular calcium ion are known to be regulatory substances whose cytoplasmic concentrations dramatically influence a variety of platelet functions.[11]

Cyclic AMP

Cyclic AMP (cAMP) is generated from ATP by the enzyme adenyl cyclase (Fig. 6–5). This enzyme is located in the platelet cell membrane

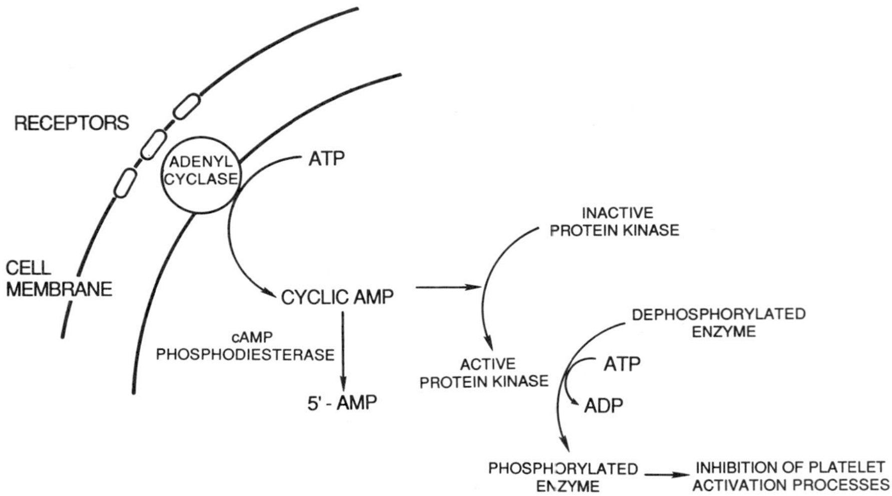

Figure 6–5. Cyclic AMP (cAMP) serves as an intracellular messenger coupling stimulus-receptor interaction at the cell surface with the intracellular regulatory and metabolic processes. cAMP is generated from ATP by the enzyme adenyl cyclase at the cytoplasmic face of the platelet cell membrane. The enzyme is closely related to membrane surface receptors that regulate its activity. Adenyl cyclase activity is either promoted or inhibited by extracellular stimuli through their interaction with specific receptors.

Released into the cytoplasm, cAMP activates a cAMP-dependent protein kinase that catalyzes the phosphorylation of substrate proteins. Phosphorylation of enzymes alters their activities, increasing the activity of some enzymes, while inhibiting others. In the platelet, protein kinase–induced phosphorylation specifically inhibits enzymes catalyzing the metabolic processes that cause platelet activation. Intracellular levels of cAMP are reduced by its degradation to 5′-AMP by cyclic nucleotide phosphodiesterases.

and is closely associated with the membrane surface receptors. The generation of cAMP occurs on the cytoplasmic side of the plasma membrane, and the cAMP is released into the cell interior. Within the cell, cAMP may be either degraded to 5′-AMP by one of two cyclic nucleotide phosphodiesterases or bound to a variety of proteins, including cAMP-dependent protein kinase activation. The activated protein kinase acts together with ATP to phosphorylate substrate proteins, which then act to retard the activation process. Specifically, cAMP in the platelet inhibits phospholipase activation and thereby inhibits the liberation of arachidonic acid from membrane phospholipids.[12–14] Furthermore, cAMP stimulates a calcium pump that lowers intracellular calcium levels and impairs calcium-dependent events such as phospholipase activation and microfilament contraction.[15] Finally, cAMP inhibits the conversion of arachidonic acid into prostaglandin endoperoxides by inhibiting cyclo-oxygenase.[16] Thus, increasing levels of cAMP in the platelet inhibit the platelet activation sequence at numerous steps which include, at least, platelet shape change, granule secretion, and prostaglandin synthesis.

Platelet cAMP levels are regulated by membrane-bound adenyl cyclases and two intracellular phosphodiesterases. Several of the agonists triggering platelet activation bind to specific membrane receptors, inhibiting adenyl cyclase activity and, as a result, reducing cAMP production. The reduced levels of cAMP promote the platelet activation process. Conversely, stimulation of adenyl cyclase activity produces an increase in intracellular cAMP levels, which in turn exert inhibitory effects on the platelet activation sequence. Several prostaglandins act at platelet membrane receptors to stimulate adenyl cyclase activity, increase cAMP levels, and thus inhibit platelet function. cAMP levels may also be increased and platelet function retarded by inhibition of platelet cyclic nucleotide phosphodiesterases. Inhibition of these enzymes slows cAMP degradation, allowing intracellular levels to increase (Fig. 6–5).

Intracellular Calcium

A rise in intracellular calcium concentration may be the final common pathway mediating platelet granule secretion.[11, 17–19] The rise in cytoplasmic calcium results partially from an increase in permeability and the influx of calcium across the plasma membrane, but primarily from the release of calcium from intracellular storage sites in the dense tubular system. Calcium is believed to trigger the release reaction by promoting platelet microfilament contraction, which forces secretory granules to the center of the cell, where they fuse with the surface-connecting open canalicular system.[20] Calmodulin is a low molecular weight calcium-binding protein that is associated with intracellular calcium and is present in platelets.[19, 21] This protein may regulate a variety of platelet enzymes, including the cyclic nucleotide phosphodiesterases, adenyl cyclase, protein kinase, and phospholipases A_2 and C. Thus, factors that alter calcium availability in the platelet will regulate platelet responsiveness to triggering stmuli.

Summary

Although our understanding of the stimulus-response coupling in the platelet is incomplete, it is clear that cAMP, intracellular calcium, and at least three specific stimulus-response coupling pathways are involved. The variety of intracellular effects of cAMP and calcium suggests that these intracellular regulators have central roles in determining the extent to which platelets respond to triggering agonists. It is also apparent that the actions of each of the known regulators of platelet function are interrelated and, to a certain degree, all inseparable. For example, cAMP regulates cytoplasmic calcium levels and, therefore, calcium-mediated processes, while intracellular calcium levels influence, in part, cAMP concentrations by mediating the activity of the enzymes that generate and degrade cAMP.

Knowledge of platelet structure and function provides a basis for understanding platelet behavior in "unphysiological" circumstances, including those associated with cardiac surgery. Comparision of platelet reactivity during extracorporeal circulation with that occurring under physiological conditions provides insight into mechanisms of platelet behavior in all situations. Furthermore, this knowledge permits us to understand how certain pharmacological agents may interfere with platelet function.

PLATELET FUNCTION DURING CARDIOPULMONARY BYPASS

During CPB, quantitative and qualitative alterations in platelets occur as the result of interactions between the platelets and synthetic surfaces of the extracorporeal circuit, air-blood interfaces, and other factors.

Platelets and Synthetic Surfaces

Platelet contact with synthetic surfaces initiates platelet behavior similar to that promoted by weak soluble agonists as described above.[22] Platelet shape change, adhesion, aggregation, and granule secretion occur. The exposure of blood to the synthetic surface results in a deposition of blood proteins at the blood-surface interface.[23] This protein layer consists largely of fibrinogen and provides a surface conducive to platelet adhesion and aggregation. Fibrinogen binds to fibrinogen receptors exposed on activated platelets. It is an essential co-factor for platelet adhesion and is required for platelet aggregation.[24–26] Initially, platelets conveyed to the surface by interactions with tumbling red blood cells adhere to the surface and undergo shape change and degranulation. Subsequently, arriving platelets aggregate, extending the evolving platelet thrombus.

In Vitro Simulated Extracorporeal Circulation with a Membrane Oxygenator

The largest area of synthetic surface in the extracorporeal circuit is the membrane oxygenator. The behavior of platelets and synthetic surfaces may be examined during simulated in vitro extracorporeal circulation with a membrane oxygenator. In vitro systems have an advantage over the test systems that employ an animal model in that the use of human blood circumvents the problems of species variability[27] and that the platelets and their release components are not diluted or cleared during an experimental trial, as they are with in vivo models.

When human blood anticoagulated with heparin is recirculated at 37° C in vitro in a circuit containing a membrane oxygenator, the circulating platelet count declines to approximately 20 per cent of initial levels within two minutes and slowly increases over the next several hours.[28] An element of platelet loss during in vitro recirculation is clearly related to platelet adhesion at the surface interface as visualized by scanning electron microscopy.[28] Platelet-to-platelet interactions with aggregate formation occur in the circulating blood and also contribute to the temporary loss of platelets.

Prior exposure of the synthetic surfaces to albumin decreases the affinity of that surface for platelets and is sufficient to prevent a decline in the circulating platelet count for up to six hours. The albumin adsorption reduces platelet granule release and largely preserves the functional and morphological integrity of the platelets.[29] Surface-adsorbed albumin may reduce platelet adhesion by limiting the availability of binding sites on the synthetic surface for fibrinogen. Alternatively, albumin may bind the products of arachidonic acid metabolism, preventing platelet recruitment.

The platelet-specific protein, low affinity platelet factor 4 (LA-PF4), may be used as a sensitive indicator of the platelet release reaction in the in vitro circuit. During in vitro circulation, plasma levels of LA-PF4 rise during the first several minutes and reach approximately 50 per cent of releasable LA-PF4 within one hour.[28] Release of dense granules presumably occurs also, since there are no precedents for release of LA-PF4 without concomitant release of dense granule contents. This is consistent with the observation made by transmission electron microscopy that circulating platelets removed from the in vitro circuit appear degranulated (Fig. 6–6*A*).[28]

The mechanism by which the platelet release reaction is triggered in the in vitro circuit is not clear. It is known that when platelets are challenged by soluble aggregating agents, the release reaction proceeds by at least three pathways of the stimulus-response coupling described above. While thromboxane synthesis has been detected during experimental extracorporeal circulation and correlates with the platelet-release reaction, the facts that the release reaction is only partially inhibited by aspirin and that the release of platelet secretory proteins actually precedes the onset of detectable thromboxane synthesis suggest that thromboxane-independent pathways are also operative.[30]

Prostaglandin I_2(PGI_2) (prostacyclin) is a potent platelet inhibitor synthesized by vascular endothelial cells. PGI_2 functions as an antithrom-

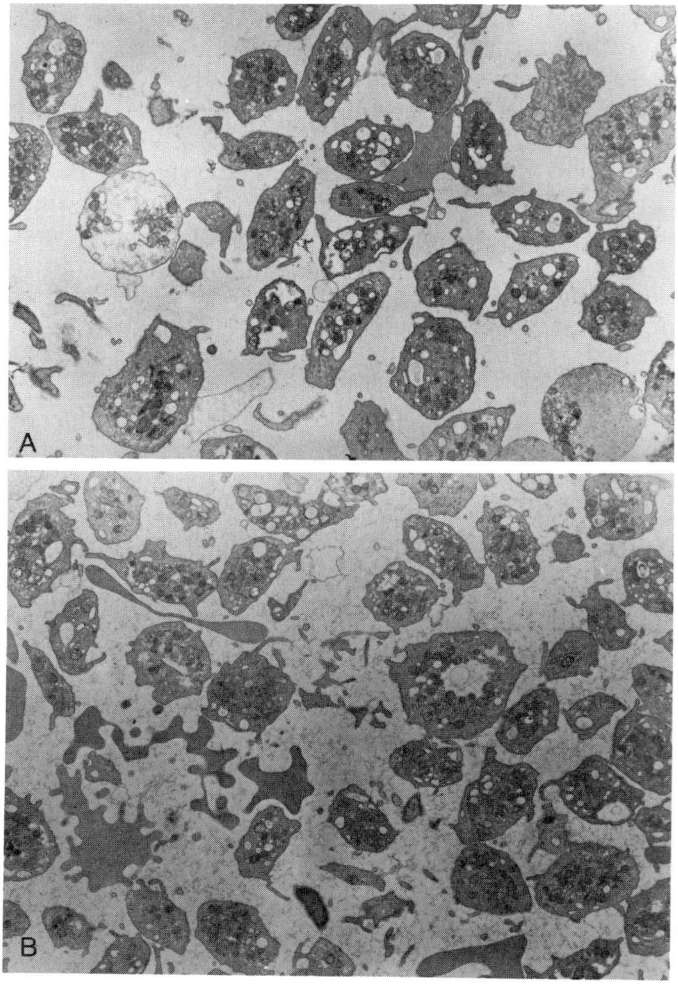

Figure 6–6. Morphological alterations in human platelets separated from blood after two hours of recirculation in an in vitro extracorporeal circuit with a membrane oxygenator observed by electron microscopy. Prior to recirculation, iloprost (2 ng/ml) was added to the circuit in which the platelets in *B* were circulated. Iloprost stimulates platelet adenyl cyclase, thereby increasing intracellular cAMP levels. Thus, this prostanoid inhibits platelet activation. Platelets in *A* were not treated with iloprost before recirculation.

A large fraction of the normally functioning platelets *(A)* demonstrate shape change with pseudopod formation and loss of cytoplasmic granules. Platelet activation occurred at the synthetic surface in the extracorporeal circuit.

Platelets recirculated with iloprost *(B)* demonstrate preserved morphology. Some pseudopod formation is seen in the inhibited platelets and occurs as an artifact of the platelet separation process. Iloprost-induced platelet inhibition prevents the occurrence of activation at synthetic surfaces and the associated morphological platelet alterations.

botic agent by stimulating platelet adenyl cyclase, resulting in an increase in intracellular cAMP. Thus, adding PGI_2 to an in vitro circuit reconstitutes one of the antithrombogenic characteristics of intact vascular endothelium. In fact, PGI_2 added to the venous reservoir of the perfusion circuit prior to recirculation completely prevents adverse platelet-surface interactions during simulated extracorporeal circulation.[29]

In Vitro Simulated Extracorporeal Circulation with a Bubble Oxygenator

During extracorporeal circulation with a bubble oxygenator, morphological and functional platelet alterations are induced as a result of platelet interaction with air-blood interfaces. These alterations occur in addition to those induced by platelet interactions at synthetic surfaces. At air-blood interfaces, platelets probably adhere to plasma protein films containing fibrinogen similar to those that occur at blood-synthetic surface interfaces. Furthermore, blood-gas interfaces have long been known to denature plasma proteins, and the mechanical destruction of large numbers of platelets occurs at the air interface.

During in vitro extracorporeal circulation with a bubble oxygenator, the circulating platelet count declines, but more gradually than during circulation with a membrane oxygenator. Platelet granule release is pronounced, although not quite as extensive as in the membrane oxygenator circuit.[31] These differences presumably reflect the fact that the bubble oxygenator contains less synthetic surface area for platelet-surface interaction. In the bubble oxygenator circuit, however, there is no evidence of return of platelets to circulation, presumably reflecting platelet destruction.[32, 33] Methods that prevent platelet activation at synthetic surfaces (e.g., albumin adsorption, PGI_2 platelet inhibition) are only partially protective during extracorporeal circulation with bubble oxygenators. The incomplete preservation of platelet function resulting from inhibition of platelet-synthetic surface interaction and the failure of platelets to return to circulation after extracorporeal perfusion with a bubble oxygenator indicates that the platelet-air interface in the bubble oxygenator probably induces a direct platelet injury that is superimposed upon the one that accrues from platelet-surface interaction.

In Vivo Cardiopulmonary Bypass

Hemodilution is a major factor causing a decrease in the platelet count during clinical, in vivo CPB.[34, 35] During in vivo extracorporeal circulation with membrane oxygenators in humans, a decline in the platelet count corrected for hemodilution is also noted to occur.[36] The reduction in corrected platelet count reflects the occurrence of platelet aggregation induced by platelet-surface interactions. In contrast, in bubble oxygenator systems, the decline in the circulating platelet count is largely due to dilution.[36–38] This difference may be due to the reduced surface area of the bubble oxygenators.

The release reaction with secretion of platelet granule contents has been documented in vivo during extracorporeal perfusion with membrane and bubble oxygenator systems in experimental animals and humans by measurement of plasma levels of the specific proteins released from the platelet granules.[36, 39] Measured increases of PF4, LA-PF4, and beta thromboglobulin (alpha granule secretory products) occur. Presumably dense granule release occurs also, but the available data are conflicting.[37, 40]

Qualitative alterations in platelet function accompany quantitative changes following in vivo extracorporeal circulation.[36, 37, 39, 41] These platelets have a diminished sensitivity to triggering agonists and, therefore, an impaired capacity for activation and function. The platelets demonstrate reduced affinity for glass beads and a decline in reactivity when challenged by soluble agonists such as ADP and epinephrine in an aggregometer. These functional defects persist for several hours and probably contribute to the prolongation of the postoperative bleeding time observed after extracorporeal perfusion with both bubble and membrane oxygenator systems.

The precise pathological defect responsible for the resulting platelet dysfunction remains incompletely defined. The relative contributions of activation at the synthetic surface versus platelet-to-platelet interaction (with aggregate formation) to the subsequent functional defect(s) observed are, likewise, unclear. The available evidence seems to indicate that the minority of platelets are fully activated, but the majority of platelets circulate with reduced function.[37] Three hypotheses have been advanced to explain the functional defect in the circulating platelets.[22, 42] The defect may be due to the partial depletion of granule stores resulting from alpha and dense granule release, the transient occurrence of a circualting functional platelet inhibitor, or a reversible platelet membrane abnormality producing alterations in receptors for triggering agonists.[43]

In addition to the extracorporeal circuit and oxygenator, other factors contribute to the quantitative and qualitative platelet disturbances observed following in vivo CPB. Hypothermia contributes to platelet dysfunction following CPB. Transient thrombocytopenia results from sequestration of platelets when body temperature decreases below 25° C,[44] and in vitro aggregation is abolished below 33° C.[45] Platelet dysfunction after hypothermic CPB has been related to the degree of hypothermia.[46] Cardiotomy suction systems, by returning blood from the operative field, provide blood-gas and blood-tissue interfaces at which platelet activation and injury occur. The volume and percentage of blood aspirated by cardiotomy suction correlate directly with platelet loss.[47, 48] Filters are included in the perfusion circuit to reduce the number of circulating microaggregates. They may, however, paradoxically contribute to the formation of platelet aggregates by providing surfaces for platelet activation and/or destruction and contribute in part to the relative increase in the number of circulating altered platelets.[49] Other possible causes of thrombocytopenia or platelet dysfunction following CPB are platelet aggregation induced by pulmonary artery catheters, heparin, protamine, heparin-protamine complexes, and ADP released from hemolyzed red blood cells (RBC's). The intravenous injection of protamine after CPB reduces platelet counts by one third within minutes.[50] This effect is transient, lasting less than one hour, and may result from temporary sequestration of platelets in the liver.

PHARMACOLOGICAL PRESERVATION OF PLATELET FUNCTION

No completely blood-compatible synthetic surfaces exist. The observation that artificial surfaces and soluble agonists initiate similar pathways of platelet activation, however, suggests that temporary reversible platelet inhibition during contact with the synthetic surface might represent a practical alternative to the elusive goal of designing a nonthrombogenic surface.

Achieving effective temporary platelet inhibition useful in cardiovascular surgery requires that two criteria be met: (1) that platelet inhibition be relatively complete in extent and (2) that it be reversible. The achievement of complete platelet inhibition is complicated by the number of intracellular mechanisms involved in the platelet activation sequence and their complex interrelationships. Because the release reaction and secondary aggregation triggered by extracorporeal circulation occurs by at least three intracellular triggering mechanisms, inhibition of a single mechanism will produce some attenuation in platelet reaction, but the inhibition will be incomplete in effect. Complete platelet inhibition probably requires interruption of a central intracellular regulating mechanism, i.e., a common denominator, in the platelet activation process.

Pharmacological inhibitors of platelet function are currently classified by their mechanisms of action (Table 6–3). Agents may impede platelet function by (1) inhibiting cyclo-oxygenase, (2) increasing intracellular cAMP levels through stimulation of adenyl cyclase activity or inhibition of cAMP phosphodiesterases, or (3) unknown mechanisms.

Cyclo-oxygenase Inhibition

Aspirin, indomethacin, and nonsteroidal anti-inflammatory agents inhibit cyclo-oxygenase, blocking the conversion of arachidonic acid to

TABLE 6–3. DRUGS THAT IMPAIR PLATELET FUNCTION (LISTED BY MECHANISM OF ACTION)

- A. Drugs Inhibiting Qualitative Platelet Function
  - 1. Cyclo-oxygenase Inhibition
    - Aspirin
    - Indomethacin
    - Nonsteroidal anti-inflammatory agents
      - Ibuprofen
      - Mefenamic acid
      - Naproxen
      - Phenylbutazone
      - Sulfinpyrazone
  - 2. Elevation of Intracellular Cyclic AMP
    - Adenyl cyclase stimulation
      - Adenosine
      - Beta-adrenergic agonists, e.g., isoproterenol
      - Iloprost
      - PGI_2, PGE_1, PGD_1, PGD_2
    - Cyclic AMP phosphodiesterase inhibition
    - Dipyridamole
    - Methylxanthines
      - Aminophylline
      - Caffeine
      - Theophylline
    - Papaverine
  - 3. Unclear Mechanisms of Qualitative Inhibition
    - Antihistamines (H_1 receptor blockers)
      - Diphenhydramine
    - Beta-adrenergic antagonists
      - Propranolol
    - Calcium channel blockers
      - Diltiazem
      - Verapamil
    - Local anesthetics
    - Penicillins and semisynthetic penicillins
      - Carbenicillin
      - Nafcillin
      - Penicillin G
      - Ticarcillin
    - Phenothiazines
      - Chlorpromazine
      - Trifluoperazine
    - Tricyclic antidepressants
      - Amitryptyline
      - Doxepin
      - Impramine
    - Vascular smooth muscle relaxants
      - Hydralazine
      - Nitroglycerin
      - Sodium nitroprusside
- B. Drugs Causing Thrombocytopenia
  - 1. Antibiotics
    - Cephalothin
    - Gentamycin
    - Sulfonamides
  - 2. Diuretics
    - Acetazolamide
    - Chlorothiazide
    - Ethacrynic acid
    - Furosemide
  - 3. Gold salts
  - 4. Heparin
  - 5. Protamine
  - 6. Quinidine

cyclic endoperoxides and their derivatives, including thromboxane A_2. Aspirin acts irreversibly by acetylating cyclo-oxygenase.[51] The duration of aspirin's antiplatelet effects is for the lifespan of the platelet, 10 to 14 days. The drug is widely employed, often in conjunction with dipyridamole, a cAMP phosphodiesterase inhibitor, in the management of thromboembolic vascular disorders, including coronary artery disease. Thus, many patients present for cardiac surgery with irreversible platelet inhibition due to aspirin therapy.

Despite its ability to prolong bleeding time and its efficacy in the control of certain thromboembolic disorders, aspirin provides incomplete inhibition of platelet activation during extracorporeal circulation.[30] The degree of platelet inhibition achieved during CPB with cyclo-oxygenase inhibitors is incomplete, since arachidonate metabolism is only one of several mechanisms regulating platelet responsiveness. In any case, the use of these agents for this purpose is impractical, since their duration of action is uncontrollably prolonged and may itself contribute to postoperative platelet dysfunction.

Elevation of Intracellular Cyclic AMP

The multiple regulatory actions of the intracellular mediator, cAMP, suggest that pharmacological elevation of platelet cAMP levels may provide effective platelet inhibition during extracorporeal circulation.

Phosphodiesterase inhibition by dipyridamole (Persantine) results in an increase in intracellular cAMP, inhibition of in vitro platelet aggregation, and prolongation of platelet lifespan in vivo.[52] Dipyridamole is frequently administered in conjunction with aspirin for their synergistic effects on platelet function.[53] It is somewhat more effective than aspirin in preserving platelet function during extracorporeal circulation in experimental animals and humans.[54] The potency of dipyridamole is insufficient, however, to completely prevent platelet reactivity during extracorporeal circulation, and its duration of action cannot be controlled. Nevertheless, a variety of phosphodiesterase inhibitors are in clinical use and may be expected to impair platelet function (Table 6–3).

The most potent inhibitors of platelet function are prostaglandins PGE_1, PGI_2, and PGD_2, which increase intracellular cAMP levels by adenyl cyclase stimulation. PGE_1 was the first prostaglandin studied in regard to complete therapeutic platelet inhibition, but it was found to be too vasoactive for clinical use. PGI_2 (prostacyclin) is a naturally occurring prostaglandin that is a more potent inhibitor than PGE_1 but is also very vasoactive and chemically unstable. Prostanoids are synthetic substances with many of the characteristics of prostaglandins. A newly developed prostanoid, iloprost (Berlex Laboratories, Inc., Cedar Knolls, NJ), is a stable analogue of prostacyclin. It is 10 times as potent, chemically stable, and less vasoactive than its parent compound with a plasma half-life of approximately 15 minutes.[55] In contrast to aspirin, therefore, this prostanoid inhibits platelet activation by modifying levels of a vital intracellular mediator; in contrast to aspirin and dipyridamole it is of short duration of action; and in contrast to PGE_1 and prostacyclin, it is less vasoactive and clinically applicable.

During in vitro extracorporeal circulation with a membrane oxygenator, iloprost prevents platelet granule secretion and preserves platelet count and functional and morphological integrity (Fig. 6–6).[56] Potential clinical roles for this prostanoid may exist in circumstances in which temporary, complete inhibition of platelet activation will be of benefit. The inhibition of platelet activation at synthetic surfaces during extracorporeal circulation (including the use of CPB, extracorporeal membrane oxygenation, and left ventricular assist devices) may be achieved by the continuous infusion of the drug, permitting the prompt restoration of platelet reactivity when the infusion is discontinued. The efficacy of platelet inhibition of iloprost during in vivo CPB with membrane oxygenator systems is currently under investigation. Because activation at synthetic surfaces only partially contributes to alterations in platelet function produced during extracorporeal circulation with bubble oxygenator systems, prostanoid-induced platelet inhibition will provide incomplete preservation of platelet function in this circumstance. The single approved clinical indication for administration of this prostanoid at the present time is the prevention of heparin-induced platelet activation in patients with confirmed heparin-induced thrombocytopenia (HIT) requiring heparin anticoagulation during cardiovascular surgery (see Ch. 8).

Other known adenyl cyclase stimulators in platelets include adenosine and beta-adrenergic agonists, e.g., isoproterenol. In comparision with the prostaglandins, neither adenosine nor beta agonists are potent platelet inhibitors.

Interestingly, halothane, at clinical concentrations, has been demonstrated to activate adenyl cyclase,[57] decrease in vitro platelet aggregation,[57–59] and prolong bleeding times in patients during anesthesia.[60–62] The inhibitory effect is rapidly reversed upon discontinuation of the anesthetic agent.[59] Platelet inhibition by nitrous oxide, enflurane, and isoflurane has not been demonstrated.[62] While these studies are of interest to anesthesiologists, their clinical relevance remains to be determined.

Unknown Mechanisms of Inhibition

A number of drugs impair in vitro platelet function by mechanisms that are unknown or are imprecisely defined. Some of these agents are relevant to the anesthesiologist. Sodium nitroprusside and nitroglycerin, vascular smooth muscle relaxants, are potent inhibitors of in vitro aggregation.[63–65] Whether these drugs act by inhibiting contraction of microfilaments or by other mechanisms is unknown.

Calcium channel blocking agents[66–68] reversibly inhibit platelet aggregation in vitro. They are weak inhibitors presumably because they block the transport of extracellular calcium into the platelet. Intracellular calcium derived from the dense tubular system, however, is sufficient to promote a complete release reaction.

Several drugs inhibit platelet function through a variety of effects on platelet membrane functions required for normal platelet reactivity.[69] These actions may include impairment of agonist-receptor interaction, interference with arachidonic acid cleavage from membrane phospholipids, and inhibition of calmodulin activity. Agents that depress platelet membrane function include propranolol, local anesthetics, phenothiazines, tricyclic antidepressants, H_1-receptor antihistamines, and semisynthetic penicillins.

Thus, medications with platelet inhibitory side effects (Table 6–3) are frequently prescribed for cardiac surgery patients preoperatively and are administered intraoperatively. Some of these drugs are commonly used in cardiovascular anesthesia and surgery. While varying degrees of in vitro inhibition of platelet function can be measured as a result of the medications' effects on platelets (in some instances, prolonged bleeding times may be observed), the contribution of these drugs to the intraoperative or postoperative platelet dysfunction occurring with cardiac surgery is undefined. The degree of platelet inhibition produced by these drugs is much less than that required for the purpose of platelet function preservation during extracorporeal circulation.

In addition to drug-induced inhibition of platelet function, thrombocytopenia may be associated with the administration of certain medications in the perioperative period (Table 6–3).[70] Drug-related thrombocytopenia may be immune-mediated and causes a decrease in platelet count that is generally transient and of mild clinical significance.

SUMMARY

Quantitative and qualitative platelet deficiencies are the most predictably observed defects in hemostatic function following cardiac surgery. Alterations in platelet function may result from factors that dilute the number of circulating platelets, sequester platelets from circulation, directly inhibit platelet function, trigger platelet activation, or produce other platelet injuries. Platelet activation during cardiac surgery is triggered by the fibrinogen-coated synthetic surfaces of the extracorporeal circuit. Platelet-surface interactions initiate the release reaction, and the secretory products liberated then induce platelet-to-platelet interactions, causing aggregate formation. Surface adhesion and platelet aggregation result in a reduction in the number of circulating platelets. More importantly, the platelets remaining in circulation have impaired function. The pathological mechanism explaining the qualitative platelet defect is not precisely defined.

While normal platelet function usually returns within several hours after the discontinuation of CPB, postoperative platelet dysfunction can be marked or persistent, resulting in hemorrhagic complications and reoperation. Platelet deficiencies causing excessive bleeding following cardiac surgery are especially likely when extracorporeal circulation is associated with the prolonged use of a bubble oxygenator, cardiotomy suction, or deep hypothermia. In these instances, direct and irreversible platelet injuries are superimposed upon those resulting from platelet interaction at synthetic surfaces. Additional disturbances in platelet function may originate with the preoperative use of medications with incidental antiplatelet activity and may exacerbate postoperative hemorrhage. The first line of treatment of postoperative hemorrhage should include measures that restore platelet function, including platelet transfusion.

Postoperative platelet dysfunction that results from platelet activation by synthetic surfaces in the extracorporeal circuit may be reduced by the use of drugs that effectively and temporarily inhibit platelet reactivity during CPB. A prostanoid, iloprost, is an analogue of prostacyclin that currently offers the most promise as a clinically useful inhibitor of platelet activation and as a means of preserving platelet function following extracorporeal circulation.

Acknowledgments

The authors wish to express their gratitude to Carol A. Fisher, A.B., for her valuable editorial review of the manuscript and to Ms. Carmen Herrera for her expert secretarial assistance.

References

1. Excerpted from material originally appearing in Harker L: Bleeding after cardiopulmonary bypass. N Engl J Med 314:1446–1448, 1986.
1a. Bachmann F, McKenna R, Cole ER, Najafi H: The hemostatic mechanism after open heart surgery. I. Studies on plasma coagulation factors and fibrinolysis in 512 patients after extracorporeal circulation. J Thorac Cardiovasc Surg 70:76–85, 1975.
2. Williams WJ, Beutler E, Erslev AJ, Lichtman MA (eds): Hematology (ed 3). New York, McGraw-Hill, 1983.
3. Colman RW, Hirsh J, Marder VJ, Salzman EW (eds): Hemostasis and Thrombosis. Philadelphia, JB Lippincott Company, 1982.
4. Weiss HJ: Platelet physiology and abnormalities of platelet function. N Engl J Med 293:531–541, 580–588, 1975.
5. Karpatkin S, Holmsen H: Composition of platelets. *In* Williams WJ, Beutler E, Erslev AJ, Lichtman MA (eds): Hematology (ed 3). New York, McGraw-Hill, 1983, pp 1136–1149.
6. Holmsen H: Platelet secretion. *In* Colman RW, Hirsh J, Marder VJ, Salzman EW (eds): Hemostasis and Thrombosis. Philadelphia, JB Lippincott Company, 1982, pp 390–403.
7. Verstraete M, Dejana E, Fuster V, et al.: An overview of antiplatelet and antithrombotic drugs. Haemostasis 15:89–99, 1985.
8. Rittenhouse-Simmons S, Russell FA, Deykin D: Mobilization of arachidonic acid in human platelet kinetics and Ca^{2+} dependency. Biochim Biophys Acta 488:370–380, 1977.
9. Hornstra G, Haddeman E, Don JA: Some investigations into the role of prostacyclin in thromboregulation. Thromb Res 12:367–374, 1977.
10. Packham MA, Kinlough-Rathbone RL, Reimers S, Mustard JF: Mechanisms of platelet

aggregation independent of adenosine diphosphate. *In* Silver MS, et al. (eds): Prostaglandins in Hematology. New York, Spectrum, 1977, pp 247–276.
11. Steer ML, Salzman EW: Intracellular regulatory processes in platelets. *In* Colman RW, Hirsh J, Marder VJ, Salzman EW (eds): Hemostasis and Thrombosis. Philadelphia, JB Lippincott Company, 1982, pp 486–495.
12. Gerrard JM, Peller JD, Krick TP, White JG: Cyclic AMP and platelet prostaglandin synthesis. Prostaglandins 14:39–50, 1977.
13. Lapetina EG, Schitges A, Chandrabose K: Cyclic adenosine 3′,5′-monophosphate and prostacyclin inhibit membrane phospholipase activity in platelets. Biochem Biophys Res Commun 76:828–835, 1977.
14. Minkes M, Stanford N, Chi MM-Y, et al.: Cyclic adenosine 3′,5′-monophosphate inhibits the availability of arachidonate to prostaglandin synthetase in human platelet suspensions. J Clin Invest 59:449–454, 1977.
15. Kaser-Glanzmann R, Jakabova M, George JN, Luscher EF: Stimulation of calcium uptake in platelet membrane vesicles by adenosine 3′,5′-cyclic monophosphate and protein kinase. Biochim Biophys Acta 466:429–440, 1977.
16. Malmsten C, Granstrom E, Samuelsson B: Cyclic AMP inhibits synthesis of prostaglandin endoperoxide (PGG_2) in human platelets. Biochem Biophys Res Commun 68:569–576, 1976.
17. Murer EH, Stewart GJ, Rausch MA, Day JH: Calcium ionophore A23187 (Eli Lilly): Effect on platelet function, structure, and metabolism. Thromb Diath Haemorrh 34:72–82, 1975.
18. White JG, Rao GHR, Gerrard JM: Effects of the ionophore A_{23187} on blood platelets. I. Influence on aggregation and secretion. Am J Pathol 77:135–150, 1974.
19. Young NJ, Crawford N: Isolation from blood platelets and polymorphs of a Ca^{2+}-dependent regulator protein (CDR) which activates cyclic nucleotide phosphodiesterase. Thromb Haemost 42:81, 1979.
20. White JG: Electron microscopic studies of platelet secretion. *In* Spaeth TH (ed): Progress in Hemostasis and Thrombosis. Vol 2. New York, Grune & Stratton, 1974, pp 49–98.
21. Levine SN, Steiner AL, White GC: Identification and distribution of the calcium-dependent regulator protein in human platelet preparations. Thromb Haemost 42:81, 1979.
22. Addonizio VP, Colman RW: Platelets and extracorporeal circulation. Biomaterials 3:9–15, 1982.
23. Baier RE, Dutton RC: Initial events in interactions of blood with a foreign surface. J Biomed Mat Res 3:191–206, 1969.
24. Mason RG, Read MS, Brinkhaus KM: Effect of fibrinogen concentration on platelet adhesion to glass. Proc Soc Exp Biol Med 137:680–682, 1971.
25. Mustard JF, Packham MA, Kinloug RI, et al.: Fibrinogen and ADP-induced platelet aggregation. Blood 52:453–466, 1978.
26. Zucker MB, Vroman L: Platelet adhesion induced by fibrinogen adsorbed onto glass. Proc Soc Exp Biol Med 131:318–320, 1969.
27. Addonizio VP: Species effects in testing materials and cardiovascular devices in experimental animals. *In* Guidelines for Blood-Materials Interactions. National Heart, Lung, and Blood Institute. NIH Publication No. 85–2185, July 1985.
28. Addonizio VP Jr, Macarak RJ, Colman RW, et al.: Preservation of human platelets with prostaglandin E_1 during in vitro simulation of cardiopulmonary bypass. Circ Res 44:350–357, 1979.
29. Addonizio VP Jr., Macarak J, Nicolaou KC, et al.: Effects of prostacyclin and albumin on platelet loss during in vitro simulation of extracorporeal circulation. Blood 53:1033–1042, 1979.
30. Addonizio VP Jr, Smith JB, Guiod LR, et al.: Thromboxane synthesis and platelet protein release during simulated extracorporeal circulation. Blood 54:171–176, 1979.
31. Addonizio VP Jr, Strauss JF III, Colman RW, Edmunds LH Jr: Effects of prostaglandin E_1 on platelet loss during in vivo and in vitro extracorporeal circulation with a bubble oxygenator. J Thorac Cardiovasc Surg 77:119–126, 1979.
32. van den Dungen JJ, Karliczek GF, Brenken U, et al.: Clinical study of blood trauma during perfusion with membrane and bubble oxygenators. J Thorac Cardiovasc Surg 83:108–116, 1982.

33. Peterson KA, Dewangee MK, Kaye MP: Fate of indium 111-labeled platelets during cardiopulmonary bypass performed with membrane and bubble oxygenators. J Thorac Cardiovasc Surg 84:39–43, 1982.
34. Hope AF, Heyns A duP, Lotter MG, et al.: Kinetics and sites of sequestration of indium 111-labeled human platelets during cardiopulmonary bypass. J Thorac Cardiovasc Surg 81:880–886, 1981.
35. Mammen EF, Koets MH, Washington BC, et al.: Hemostasis changes during cardiopulmonary bypass surgery. Semin Thromb Hemost 11:281–292, 1985.
36. Edmunds LH Jr, Ellison N, Colman RW, et al.: Platelet function during open heart surgery: Comparison of membrane and bubble oxygenators. J Thorac Cardiovasc Surg 83:805–812, 1982.
37. Harker LA, Malpass TW, Branson HE, et al.: Mechanisms of abnormal bleeding in patients undergoing cardiopulmonary bypass: Acquired transient platelet dysfunction associated with selective alpha granule release. Blood 56:824–834, 1980.
38. McKenna R, Bachman F, Whitaker B, et al.: The hemostatic mechanism after open heart surgery. J Thorac Cardiovasc Surg 70:298–304, 1975.
39. Addonizio VP Jr, Strauss JF III, Macarack EJ, et al.: Preservation of platelet number and function with prostaglandin E_1 during total cardiopulmonary bypass in rhesus monkeys. Surgery 83:619–625, 1978.
40. Beurling-Harbury C, Galvan CA: Acquired decrease in platelet secretory ADP associated with increased postoperative bleeding in post-cardiopulmonary bypass patients and in patients with severe valvular heart disease. Blood 52:13–23, 1978.
41. Tamari Y, Aledort L, Puzskin E, et al.: Functional changes in platelets during extracorporeal circulation. Ann Thorac Surg 19:639–647, 1975.
42. Edmunds LH, Addonizio VP: Platelet physiology during cardiopulmonary bypass. *In* Utley JR (ed): Pathophysiology and Techniques of Cardiopulmonary Bypass. Vol. 1. Baltimore, Williams & Wilkins, 1982, pp 106–119.
43. Musial J, Niewiarowski S, Hershock D, et al.: Loss of fibrinogen receptors from the platelet surface during simulated extracorporeal circulation. J Lab Clin Med 105:514–522, 1985.
44. Aster RH: Thrombocytopenia due to sequestration of platelets. *In* Williams WJ, Beutler E, Erslev AJ, Lichtman MA (eds): Hematology (ed 3). New York, McGraw-Hill, 1983, pp 1338–1340.
45. Holmsen H, Karpatkin S: Metabolism of platelets. *In* Williams WJ, Beutler E, Erslev AJ, Lichtman MA (eds): Hematology (ed 3). New York, McGraw-Hill, 1983, pp 1157–1176.
46. Thomas R, Hessel EA, Harker LA, et al.: Platelet function during and after deep surface hypothermia. J Surg Res 31:314–318, 1981.
47. Edmunds LH Jr, Saxena NC, Hillyer P, Wilson TJ: Relationship between platelet count and cardiotomy suction return. Ann Thorac Surg 25:306–310, 1978.
48. Morris KN, Kinross FM, Stirling GR: Hemolysis of blood in the pericardium: The major source of plasma hemoglobin during total body perfusion. J Thorac Cardiovasc Surg 49:250, 1965.
49. Dutton RC, Edmunds LH Jr, Hutchinson JC, Rose BB: Platelet aggregate emboli produced in patients during cardiopulmonary bypass with membrane and bubble oxygenators and blood filters. J Thorac Cardiovasc Surg 67:258–265, 1974.
50. Heyns A duP: Kinetics and in vivo redistribution of 111 indium-labeled human platelets after intravenous protamine sulfate. Thromb Haemost 44:65, 1980.
51. Weiss HJ, Aledort IM: Impaired platelet-connective tissue reaction in man after aspirin ingestion. Lancet 1:495, 1967.
52. Horch U, Kadatz R, Kopitar Z, Weisenberger H: Pharmacology of dipyridamole and its derivatives. Thromb Diath Haemorrh 42(Suppl):253, 1970.
53. Raja SM, Penny AF, Crow MJ, et al.: The interaction of varying doses of dipyridamole and acetyl salicylic acid on the inhibition of platelet functions and their effect on bleeding time. Br J Clin Pharmacol 8:483–489, 1979.
54. Nuutinen LS, Mononen P: Dipyridamole and thrombocyte count in open heart surgery. J Thorac Cardiovasc Surg 70:707–711, 1975.
55. Fisher CA, Kappa JR, Sinha AK, et al.: Comparison of equimolar concentrations of

iloprost, prostacyclin, and prostaglandin E_1 on human platelet function. J Lab Clin Med 109:184–190, 1987.
56. Addonizio VP, Fisher CA, Jenkin BK, et al.: Iloprost (ZK 36374), a stable analogue of prostacyclin, preserves platelets during simulated extracorporeal circulation. J Thorac Cardiovasc Surg 89:926–933, 1985.
57. Walter F, Vulliemoz Y, Verosky M, Triner L: Effects of halothane on the cyclic 3′,5′-adenosine monophosphate enzyme system in humana platelets. Anesth Analg 59:856–861, 1980.
58. Ueda I: The effects of volatile general anesthetics on adenosine diphosphate-induced platelet aggregation. Anesthesiology 34:405–408, 1971.
59. Dalsgaard-Nielsen J: Effects of halothane on platelet function. Thromb Haemost 44:143, 1980.
60. Dalsgaard-Nielsen J, Risbo A, Simmelkjaer P, Gormsen J: Impaired platelet aggregation and increased bleeding time during general anesthesia with halothane. Br J Anaesth 53:1039–1042, 1981.
61. Stengert K: Halothane-induced platelet dysfunction. Anesth Analg 61:217, 1982.
62. Fyman PN, Triner L, Schranz H, et al.: Effect of volatile anaesthetics and nitrous oxide-fentanyl anaesthesia on bleeding time. Br J Anaesth 56:1197–1200, 1984.
63. Glusa E, Markwardt F, Sturzebecker J: Effects of sodium nitroprusside and other pentanitrosyl complexes on platelet aggregation. Haemostasis 3:249–256, 1974.
64. Mehta J, Mehta P: Comparative effects of nitroprusside and nitroglycerin on platelet aggregation in patients with heart failure. J Cardiovasc Pharmacol 2:25–33, 1980.
65. Saxon A, Kattlove HE: Platelet inhibition by sodium nitroprusside, a smooth muscle inhibitor. Blood 47:957, 1976.
66. Addonizio VP, Fisher CA, Strauss JF, Edmunds LH: Inhibition of human platelet function by verapamil. Thromb Res 28:545–556, 1982.
67. Kiyomoto A, Saski Y, Odawara A, et al.: Inhibition of platelet aggregation by diltiazem: Comparison with verapamil and nifedipine and inhibitory potencies of diltiazem metabolites. Circ Res 53(Suppl 1):115–119, 1983.
68. Addonizio VP, Fisher CA, Strauss JF III, et al.: Effects of verapamil and diltiazem on human platelet function. Am J Physiol 25:H366-HL371, 1986.
69. Mills DCB: The mechanism of action of antiplatelet drugs. *In* Colman RW, Hirsh J, Marder VJ, Salzman EW (eds): Hemostasis and Thrombosis. Philadelphia, JB Lippincott Company, 1982, pp 1058–1067.
70. Aster RH: Thrombocytopenia due to enhanced platelet destruction. *In* Williams WJ, Beutler E, Erslev AJ, Lichtman MA (eds): Hematology (ed 3). New York, McGraw-Hill 1983, pp 1298–1338.

CHAPTER 7

PLATELET TRANSFUSION*

LINDA C. STEHLING

Patients undergoing cardiopulmonary bypass (CPB) exhibit decreased platelet counts and thrombocytopathy intra- and postoperatively.[5, 17, 18, 26, 35] The exact etiology of the platelet defects remains unclear, and correlations between laboratory and clinical findings are unpredictable.[14, 18, 27] There is no single therapeutic approach to patients with bleeding presumed due to platelet abnormalities, necessitating a logical plan of evaluation and management for each patient. Platelets should be administered only when indicated, not according to a protocol based on surgical procedure, length of CPB, number of units of red blood cells (RBC's) transfused, or isolated laboratory parameters. Frequent evaluation of the patient and the response to therapy is essential in determining appropriate treatment.

PATHOPHYSIOLOGY OF THROMBOCYTOPENIA AND THROMBOCYTOPATHY

Thrombocytopenia

Hemodilution is usually considered the major factor responsible for a decrease in platelet count during CPB.[20, 26] The volume of priming solution influences the degree of hemodilution, and a platelet count decrease of approximately 30 per cent can be anticipated owing to hemodilution. However, a relatively larger decrease is usually seen in the platelet count than in the hematocrit.[26] The platelet count decreases within minutes of initiation of CPB. Further decreases of lesser magnitude

*This investigation was supported in part by a Public Health Transfusion Medicine Award (No. 1 KO7-HLO1257) from the National Heart Lung and Blood Institute, NIH.

may continue for 24 to 48 hours. The count usually returns to the preoperative level within one week.[32] Disaggregation of platelet aggregates formed during CPB may contribute to the recovery of the platelet count.[1]

Platelet destruction occurs as a result of turbulent flow and shear stresses generated during CPB. Platelets also adhere to the surface of the perfusion apparatus.[1, 5, 17] Variations in platelet counts reported by different investigators are related in part to differences in types of oxygenators and pumps, suctioning techniques, flow rates, degree of hypothermia, and bypass time. Other possible causes of thrombocytopenia are aggregation of platelets by heparin, protamine, heparin-protamine complexes, or ADP released from hemolyzed RBC's, and disseminated intravascular coagulation (DIC). The platelet counts reported by numerous investigators are quite variable (Table 7–1). However, the mean values all exceed 50,000/μl. Most importantly, the presence of clinically abnormal bleeding does not usually correlate with platelet counts obtained in the preoperative, intraoperative, or postoperative periods. The platelet count is only rarely low enough to explain abnormal bleeding following CPB. Alterations in platelet function are far more important in determining postoperative bleeding in these patients.

Thrombocytopathy

Transient impairment of platelet function occurs as a result of platelet activation during passage of platelets through the CPB apparatus. It is generally agreed that the degree of platelet dysfunction is proportional to the duration of bypass and probably related to the degree of hypothermia.[17, 40] The exact nature of the impairment is unknown, but it may be due to transient depletion of a functional platelet component, generation of a labile inhibitor, or a reversible membrane abnormality.[17, 33] Platelet dysfunction parallels a demonstrable depletion of platelet-specific proteins from the platelets and their subsequent appearance in plasma. Release and partial depletion of alpha granules, but not dense granules, occur in the platelets. Normalization of platelet function parallels clearance of the platelet proteins from the plasma.[18] In most patients, platelet dysfunction reverses within a short time following discontinuation of CPB.[10, 17] When it persists, abnormal bleeding occurs.

PREOPERATIVE EVALUATION

When evaluating a patient presenting for cardiac surgery, the anesthesiologist must be careful not to focus entirely on the cardiovascular system. The patient should be questioned about events suggestive of a bleeding diathesis such as gingival bleeding with toothbrushing, easy

TABLE 7–1. PLATELET COUNTS IN PATIENTS UNDERGOING CARDIOPULMONARY BYPASS

Author/Year	No. of Patients	Platelet Count* Preop	Postop	Remarks
Marengo-Rowe, 1979[27]	774	240 ± 73†	—	
		—	133 ± 52	end bypass
Harker, 1980[18]	31	225 ± 22	—	
		—	132 ± 16	2–4 hr post–CPB no clinical bleeding, BT‡ 8.9 ± 0.6 min
	10	—	110 ± 15	2–4 hr post–CPB, clinical bleeding, BT 23.0 ± 7.5 min
Milam, 1981[30]	75	194 ± 58	—	
		—	119 ± 45.9	30 min CPB
		—	144 ± 49.9	1 hr postop
		—	156 ± 51.1	24 hr postop
		—	149 ± 48.0	48 hr postop
Simon, 1984[37]	14	222 ± 88	—	
		—	118 ± 54	end bypass
			113 ± 33	24 hr later no platelets administered
	14	220 ± 62	—	
		—	97 ± 40	end bypass
		—	130 ± 36	24 hr later platelets administered
Mammen, 1985[26]	33	243 ± 63	—	
		—	141 ± 72	during CPB
		—	120 ± 82	in ICU
		—	126 ± 79	48 hr postop
Salzman, 1986[35]	35	178 ± 63	—	
		—	117 ± 44	no treatment
	35	151 ± 61	—	
		—	96 ± 36	after DDAVP administration
Mohr, 1986[31]	41	217 ± 78	—	
		—	127 ± 43	no clinical bleeding
	10	180 ± 40	—	
		—	93 ± 22	clinical bleeding

*(× $10^2/\mu l$)
† mean ± S.D.
‡Bleeding time
The platelet counts reported by various authors vary considerably. The reader is referred to the original papers for details of the timing of laboratory determinations, clinical conditions, and therapeutic interventions.

bruising, epistaxis, or spontaneous bleeding. Inquiries into family history should include bleeding tendencies in parents, siblings, and children in order to identify hereditary disorders that may not be evident in the patient who has not experienced surgery or trauma.

The drug history is of special importance, as many patients will be taking medications that interfere with coagulation. Aspirin is the most common drug associated with platelet dysfunction. Antibiotics can also induce platelet dysfunction,[5, 17] as can beta blockers and calcium channel blocking agents,[22] nitroprusside and nitroglycerine,[24, 29, 36] antidepressants, diuretics, and even local[2] and inhalation anesthetic agents[41] (Table 7–2). Many drugs interfere with platelet function for as long as 10 to 14 days.[5]

Acquired platelet dysfunction is a feature of many systemic diseases. The anesthesiologist must be aware of the potential for abnormal bleeding in patients with uremia,[21] myeloproliferative syndromes, malignant paraproteinemias, and autoimmune disorders.[5]

The value of preoperative coagulation tests in predicting blood loss and transfusion requirements in the absence of a positive history is uncertain.[27, 39] Nevertheless, it seems reasonable to obtain a prothrombin

TABLE 7–2. DRUGS THAT MAY INDUCE PLATELET DYSFUNCTION*

Anti-inflammatory Drugs	**Respiratory Drugs**
Aspirin	Aminophylline
Ibuprofen	Isoproterenol
Indomethacin	Theophylline
Mefenamic acid	**Psychoactive Drugs**
Naproxen	Amitryptyline
Phenylbutazone	Diazepam
Sulfinpyrazone	Chlorpromazine
Antibiotics	Doxepin
Ampicillin	Imipramine
Cabenicillin	Trifluoperazine
Cephalothin	**Miscellaneous Drugs**
Gentamycin	Alcohol
Nafcillin	Diphenhydramine
Ticarcillin	Caffeine
Diuretics	Glyceryl guaiacolate
Acetazolamide	Hydrocortisone
Ethacrynic acid	Tocopherol
Furosemide	
Cardiovascular Drugs	
Dipyridamole	
Hydralazine	
Nitroglycerin	
Papaverine	
Propranolol	
Reserpine	
Verapamil	

*This is a representative list and is not all-inclusive. It should be remembered that numerous minor analgesics and over-the-counter preparations contain aspirin.

time (PT), an activated partial thromboplastin time (aPTT), and a platelet scan. A history of abnormal bleeding or ingestion of drugs known to cause platelet dysfunction is an indication for performing a bleeding time.[5, 41] Since virtually all cardiac surgery patients are taking drugs that can cause platelet dysfunction, a bleeding time is almost always indicated. If the bleeding time is normal, surgery can proceed. If the bleeding time is prolonged, and the offending drug is one such as aspirin which can be discontinued, it is best to defer surgery for at least seven days.[41] It is wise to repeat the bleeding time before scheduling surgery. When surgery cannot be postponed, platelets should be available. Many patients with prolonged bleeding times do not bleed abnormally, and the prophylactic administration of platelets to such patients is not recommended. More extensive testing may be advisable for some children, i.e., those with cyanotic heart disease or polycythemia.[34] Platelet counts are usually performed with electronic counters. Spurious results are due to platelet clumping or marked variation in platelet size. It is thus important to examine a blood smear and compare the estimated number of platelets with the reported count.[6, 7] The normal range is 150,000 to 400,000/μl. Platelet counts are less accurate in the lower range, especially below 20,000/μl. In general, abnormal bleeding does not occur if the platelet count is greater than 100,000/μl and if the platelets are normal. In fact, it is unlikely that bleeding will occur until the platelet count is below 50,000/μl.[6]

The bleeding time is defined as the time between the infliction of a standard incision and the moment at which bleeding stops. There are two techniques to measure bleeding time: the Duke technique, in which the incision is made in the earlobe, and the Ivy technique, in which the incision is usually made on the forearm.[6] The Duke method is relatively unreliable. When the Ivy method is employed, a spring-loaded device (Simplate II, manufactured by General Diagnostics, Morris Plains, NY, or Surgicutt manufactured by International Technidyne, Edison, NJ) is usually used to make one (Surgicutt) or two (Simplate II) parallel incisions 5 mm long and 1 mm deep on the volar aspect of the forearm. A blood pressure cuff is applied to the upper arm and inflated to a pressure of approximately 40 mm Hg, and the pressure is maintained during the test. Filter paper is used to blot the blood from the incisions at 30-second intervals, and the time required to stop bleeding is recorded. When the platelet count is between 10,000 and 100,000/μl, the bleeding time and platelet count are linearly related. That relationship is expressed by the following equation:[13]

$$\text{BT (min)} = 30.5 - \frac{\text{PC } (\mu\text{l})}{3850}$$

where BT = bleeding time and PC = platelet count. However, this relationship becomes increasingly disparate following CPB.[17]

The presence of arterial and venous cannulae often preclude use of the forearm for the test. Comparison of results using the upper extremity site with the medial aspect of the calf, approximately 8 cm below the knee, indicates that the values are similar. In a recent study, the arm bleeding time was determined to be 5.6 ± 1.7 min and that of the leg 5.8 ± 2.3 min. The mean bleeding times of subjects who ingested 650 mg of aspirin was 10.2 ± 4.3 min and 9.9 ± 37 min, respectively.[19]

While the bleeding time is a rather crude test, dependent upon proper performance, it is the only readily available test of platelet function. Its use is not often practical in the operating room. However, it can be employed pre- and postoperatively. In the latter situation, the leg may be the preferred test site.

A bleeding time less than twice the upper limit of normal is usually not an indication for platelet transfusion unless there are co-existing conditions that interfere with hemostasis.[8]

Large platelets are usually considered to be more active than small ones, and the plateletcrit rather than the platelet count has been suggested as a better predictor of the risk of bleeding in patients with thrombocytopenia. The plateletcrit is calculated by multiplying the platelet count by the mean platelet volume. Preliminary studies indicate that a plateletcrit less than 0.1 per cent following CPB is an indication for platelet transfusion in patients with abnormal bleeding.[31]

Platelet aggregation studies are performed by placing platelet-rich plasma in a photometer, adding various aggregating agents, and recording the changes in light density. Epinephrine, ADP, ristocetin, collagen, arachidonic acid, and serotonin are among the aggregating agents employed. Newer instruments permit assessment of both aggregation and ATP release.[4] These complex studies require proper interpretation, and their use is generally restricted to evaluation of patients with congenital and acquired disorders of platelet function associated with normal platelet counts.

Assays of platelet factor 4, beta-thromboglobulin, and thromboxane B_2 are usually limited to research settings. They may be more useful in evaluating patients with hypercoagulable states rather than platelet function defects.[4]

POSTOPERATIVE LABORATORY STUDIES

When evaluating postoperative coagulation tests, the anesthesiologist should remember that the "normal" range for patients who have undergone CPB is not the same as that for normal volunteers or patients who have not undergone the surgery. It is "normal" for the platelet count to be decreased, the platelet function to be transiently impaired, and the bleeding time to be initially prolonged following CPB.

Trends in laboratory studies are more important than individual values. Serial values should be reviewed in light of the patient's clinical condition. When evaluating the response to platelet administration, repeat platelet counts should be obtained. The absence of an increase in platelet count one hour after platelet administration is indicative of ongoing blood loss, platelet consumption, or failure to respond to transfusion. Refractoriness is limited almost entirely to patients who have received numerous platelet transfusions in the past and have become alloimmunized, whereas fever, sepsis, and hypersplenism are associated with a shortened platelet survival.[11] Other laboratory data are necessary to confirm or refute the presence of DIC. Chest tube drainage is the best indication of the extent of bleeding.

PLATELET PRODUCTS

Platelets for transfusion are separated from whole blood or harvested from single donors by platelet pheresis. Single-donor platelets are obtained from random donors or from donors selected on the basis of HLA compatibility. Each single-donor pheresis collection provides the equivalent of the platelets from five to eight whole blood donations. Patients who receive single-donor platelets sustain less exposure to transfusion-transmitted diseases and experience reduced chances of alloimmunization. The time and equipment required for pheresis, as well as the donor commitment, limit the use of single-donor platelets almost exclusively to patients who are alloimmunized and refractory to platelet transfusion. Random- or multiple-donor platelets are relatively plentiful, since most volunteer-donor blood is fractionated.

Platelets may be stored for five days at 20 to 24° C. Constant gentle agitation during storage promotes better function of the transfused product.

Platelets are usually pooled in the blood bank when more than one unit is to be administered. Each bag of random-donor platelet should contain not less than 5.5×10^{10} platelets in 50 to 70 ml of plasma.[8] Once pooled, platelets should be transfused within six hours. They are administered through an infusion set containing a conventional 170 μ blood filter. Compatibility testing is not necessary. Platelets can be administered without regard to ABO and Rh groups unless they are heavily contaminated with RBC's. However, because some RBC's are present in platelet concentrates, it is preferable for RH-negative patients to receive Rh-negative platelets. If Rh-positive platelets are transfused to Rh-negative women with child-bearing potential, prevention of Rh immunization with Rh-immune globulin should be considered. One unit of random-donor platelets usually raises the platelet count 5,000 to 10,000/μl in the average adult. It is a common practice to infuse 1 U/10 kg of random-donor platelets.[38]

Preoperative autologous platelet pheresis and subsequent platelet transfusion have been reported in a limited number of patients undergoing CPB. While the investigators describe the procedure as safe and effective, it is unlikely that it will gain widespread acceptance.[12]

THERAPEUTIC IMPLICATIONS

It is an accepted fact that transient platelet dysfunction is associated with CPB. There are, as yet, no firm explanations for this phenomenon and no way to predict which patients will experience excessive postoperative bleeding. In addition, the definition of excessive bleeding varies. Chest tube drainage exceeding 400 ml in two hours,[3] 600 ml in the first eight hours postoperatively,[27] and 200 ml/hr in any one-hour period, or persistant drainage of 100 ml or more for a period of two hours or longer[28] has been cited as excessive bleeding by various authors. The pattern of bleeding as well as the amount must be evaluated. Is the blood loss consistent, increasing, or decreasing? Is the patient oozing from vascular cannulation sites as well as from the wound? If the only bleeding is from the chest tubes, inadequate surgical hemostasis is probable, and consideration should be given to prompt re-exploration.

Coagulation studies are most helpful when surgical bleeding is not clearly the source of the problem. Trends as well as absolute values should be evaluated in relation to the clinical situation. It cannot be overemphasized that it is the patient who must be treated. If the patient is not bleeding, even though the platelet count is low, therapy is not indicated. However, some patients bleed despite an adequate platelet count. In these circumstances, a bleeding time may be helpful. It has been suggested that a bleeding time greater than 20 minutes after administration of protamine and the presence of significant abnormal bleeding are indications for platelet administration even when the platelet count is greater than 100,000.[18]

Several investigators have demonstrated no clinical benefit from prophylactic platelet transfusion following CPB.[16, 23, 37] The Consensus Statement of the National Heart Lung and Blood Institute Conference on Platelet Transfusion Therapy is explicit in this regard: "Controlled prospective studies examining postoperative blood loss and outcome have demonstrated no correlation between platelet counts and bleeding following cardiopulmonary bypass and no detectable benefit from the prophylactic administration of platelets to such patients. The vast majority of such patients have some degree of thrombocytopenia, prolongation of the bleeding time, and continued slow bleeding. With an expected pattern of bleeding, thrombocytopenia alone is not an indication for platelet transfusion. There is no justification for prophylactic platelet administration in patients undergoing open heart surgery."[8]

Pharmacological inhibition of platelet activation during CPB is an attractive prophylactic approach. It has been demonstrated in animal studies that infusion of prostacyclin (PGI_2) will block the interaction of platelets with the artificial surfaces of the bypass apparatus, thereby preserving platelet number and function. Unfortunately, a study of the effects of prostacyclin infusion in patients undergoing CPB failed to demonstrate any beneficial effects. Moreover, the drug produced significant hypotension necessitating vasopressor therapy.[25]

Administration of desmopressin acetate (DDAVP), a synthetic vasopressin analogue, has been shown to reduce blood loss associated with CPB. The mechanism of action may be correction of platelet dysfunction[9, 35] (see Ch. 9).

SUMMARY

Thrombocytopenia per se is not an indication for platelet administration. The value of the bleeding time in predicting and evaluating postoperative blood loss and the efficacy of platelet therapy in patients with abnormal bleeding following CPB remain uncertain. Factors thought to be related to platelet dysfunction are the length of CPB, level of hypothermia, and concomitant use of semisynthetic penicillins and other drugs. The relative influence of these factors is unknown. Until the etiology of the thrombocytopathy and other contributing factors is clarified, the need for platelet administration must be determined by observation of the patient, evaluation of the available tests of coagulation, and clinical experience. There is no ideal way to administer platelets. While it often appears that cessation of bleeding coincides with the infusion of platelets, there are no studies that clearly differentiate coincidence from therapeutic effect. The risks of transfusion-transmitted diseases and alloimmunization must be weighed against the benefits of platelet administration.

Finally, transfusion practices should be periodically and systematically evaluated. Appropriately conducted, audits[15] can identify practices such as inappropriate platelet administration based solely on habit without scientific foundation.

Acknowledgment

The author wishes to acknowledge the editorial assistance offered by Mrs. Diane Coe.

References

1. Addonizio VP, Colman RW: Platelets and extracorporeal circulation. Biomaterials 3:9–15, 1982.
2. Anderson ER, Foulkes JG, Gordin DV: The effect of local anesthetics and antiarrhythmic agents on the responses of rabbit platelets to ADP and thrombin. Thromb Haemost 45:81, 1981.
3. Bachmann F, McKenna R, Cole ER, et al.: The hemostatic mechanism after open-heart surgery: I. Studies on plasma coagulation factors and fibrinolysis in 512 patients after extracorporeal circulation. J Thorac Cardiovasc Surg 70:76–85, 1975.
4. Bick RL: Disorders of Hemostasis and Thrombosis. New York, Thieme-Stratton, 1985, p 67.
5. Bick RL: Hemostasis defects associated with cardiac surgery, prosthetic devices, and other extracorporeal circuits. Semin Thromb Hemost 11:249–280, 1985.
6. Bowie EJW, Owen CA: The clinical and laboratory diagnosis of hemorrhagic disorders. *In* Miescher PA, et al. (eds): Disorders of Hemostasis. Orlando, Grune and Stratton, 1984, pp 43–72.
7. Coller BS: Disorders of platelets. *In* Miescher PA, et al. (eds): Disorders of Hemostasis. Orlando, Grune and Stratton, 1984, pp 73–176.
8. Consensus Conference: Platelet transfusion therapy. JAMA 257:1777–1780, 1987.
9. Czer L, Bateman T, Gray R, et al.: Prospective trial of DDAVP in treatment of severe platelet dysfunction and hemorrhage after cardiopulmonary bypass. Circulation 72:519, 1985.
10. Edmunds LH Jr, Ellison N, Colman RW, et al.: Platelet function during cardiac operation: Comparison membrane and bubble oxygenators. J Thorac Cardiovasc Surg 83:805–812, 1982.
11. Eisenstaedt R: Blood component therapy in the treatment of platelet disorders. Semin Hematol 23:1–7, 1986.
12. Fehir K, Jones J, Noon G, Yawn D: Preoperative autologous platelet pheresis and plasmapheresis in patients undergoing cardiopulmonary bypass procedures. Transfusion 25:580, 1985.
13. Fischbach DP, Fogdall RP: Coagulation: The Essentials. Baltimore, Williams & Wilkins, 1981, p 69.
14. Gralnick HR, Fischer RD: The hemostatic response to open-heart operations. J Thorac Cardiovasc Surg 61:909–915, 1971.
15. Grindon AJ, Tomasulo PS, Bergin JJ, et al.: The hospital transfusion committee guidelines for improving practice. JAMA 253:540–543, 1985.
16. Harding SA, Skakoor MA, Grindon AJ: Platelet support for cardiopulmonary bypass surgery. J Thorac Cardiovasc Surg 70:350–353, 1975.
17. Harker LH: Bleeding after cardiopulmonary bypass. N Engl J Med 314:1446–1447, 1986.
18. Harker LA, Malpass TW, Branson HE, et al.: Mechanism of abnormal bleeding in patients undergoing cardiopulmonary bypass: Acquired transient platelet dysfunction associated with selective a-granule release. Blood 56:824–834, 1980.
19. Hertzendorf LR, Stehling LC, Davey FR: Comparison of bleeding times performed on the arm and the leg. Am J Clin Pathol 87:393–396, 1987.
20. Hope AF, duP Heyns A, Lotter MG, et al.: Kinetics and sites of sequestration of indium 111-labeled human platelets during cardiopulmonary bypass. J Thorac Cardiovasc Surg 81:880–886, 1981.
21. Janson PA, Jubelirer SJ, Weinstein MJ, et al.: Treatment of the bleeding tendency in uremia with cryoprecipitate. N Engl J Med 303:1318–1322, 1980.
22. Kiyomoto A, Saski Y, Odawara A, et al.: Inhibition of platelet aggregation by diltiazem: Comparision with verapamil and nifedipine and inhibitory potencies of diltiazem metabolites. Circ Res 52(Suppl 1):115–119, 1983.
23. Levin J: Use of platelets in open heart surgery. Data presented at the NIH Consensus Development Conference on Platelet Transfusion Therapy, Bethesda, MD, 1986.
24. Lichtenthal PR, Rossi EC, Louis G, et al.: Dose-related prolongation of the bleeding time by intravenous nitroglycerin. Anesthesiology 64:30–33, 1985.

25. Malpass TW, Amory DW, Harker LA, et al.: The effect of prostacyclin infusion on platelet hemostatic function in patients undergoing cardiopulmonary bypass. J Thorac Cardiovasc Surg 87:550–555, 1984.
26. Mammen EF, Koets MH, Washington BC, et al.: Hemostasis changes during cardiopulmonary bypass surgery. Semin Thromb and Hemost 11:281–292, 1985.
27. Marengo-Rowe AJ, Lambert CJ, Leveson JE, et al.: The evaluation of hemorrhage in cardiac patients who have undergone extracorporeal circulation. Transfusion 19:426–433, 1979.
28. Marengo-Rowe AJ, Leveson JE: The experts opine. Surv Anesthesiol 30:377–379, 1986.
29. Mehta J, Mehta P: Comparative effects of nitroprusside and nitroglycerin on platelet aggregation in patients with heart failure. J Cardiovasc Pharmacol 2:25–33, 1980.
30. Milam JD, Austin SF, Martin RF, et al.: Alteration of coagulation and selected clinical chemistry parameters in patients undergoing open heart surgery without transfusions. Am J Clin Pathol 76:155–162, 1981.
31. Mohr R, Martinowitz U, Golan M, et al.: Platelet size and mass as an indicator for platelet transfusion after cardiopulmonary bypass. Circulation 74(Suppl III):153–158, 1986.
32. Moriau M, Masure R, Hurlet A, et al.: Haemostasis disorders in open heart surgery with extracorporeal circulation: Importance of the platelet function and the heparin neutralization. Vox Sang 32:41–51, 1977.
33. Musial J, Niewiarowski S, Hershock D, et al.: Loss of fibrinogen receptors from the platelet surface during simulated extracorporeal circulation. J Lab Clin Med 105:514–522, 1985.
34. Ramsey G, Arvan DA, Stewart S, et al.: Do preoperative laboratory tests predict blood transfusion needs in cardiac operations? J Thorac Cardiovasc Surg 85:554–569, 1983.
35. Salzman EW, Weinstein MJ, Weintraub RM, et al.: Treatment with desmospressin acetate to reduce blood loss after cardiac surgery: A double-blind randomized trial. N Engl J Med 314:1402–1406, 1986.
36. Saxon A, Kattlove HE: Platelet inhibition by sodium nitroprusside, a smooth muscle inhibitor. Blood 47:957, 1976.
37. Simon TL, Akl BF, Murphy W: Controlled trial of routine administration of platelet concentrates in cardiopulmonary bypass surgery. Ann Thorac Surg 37:359–364, 1984.
38. Snyder EL: Blood Transfusion Therapy: A Physician's Handbook. Virginia, American Association of Blood Banks, 1987, pp 14–16.
39. Suchman AL, Mushlin AI: How well does the activated partial thromboplastin time predict postoperative hemorrhage? JAMA 256:750–753, 1986.
40. Thomas R, Hessel EA III, Harker LA, et al.: Platelet function during and after deep surface hypothermia. J Surg Res 31:314–318, 1981.
41. Torosian M, Michelson EL, Morganroth J, et al.: Aspirin- and Coumadin-related bleeding after coronary-artery bypass graft surgery. Ann Intern Med 89:325–328, 1978.
42. Walter WF, Vulliemoz Y, Verosky M, et al : Effects of halothane on the cyclic 3′,5′-adenosine monophosphate enzyme system in human platelets. Anesth Analg 59:856–861, 1980.
43. Watkins J: Mechanisms and factors predisposing towards adverse response to intravenous anaesthetic substances. *In* Thornton JA (ed): Adverse Reactions to Anaesthetic Drugs. New York, Elsevier/North-Holland Biomedical, 1981, pp 137–167.

CHAPTER 8

HEPARIN-INDUCED THROMBOCYTOPENIA: Diagnosis and Management

JEFFREY R. KAPPA and V. PAUL ADDONIZIO, Jr.

Since its initial description by McLean in 1916,[1] the clinical use of heparin as an effective yet reversible anticoagulant has led to major advances in the fields of cardiac surgery, vascular surgery, nephrology, and hematology. Yet, in contrast to its fairly well-characterized effects on the coagulant proteins, the interactions between heparin and platelets remain incompletely defined. Indeed, some of these interactions can be potentially detrimental.

A mild, transient decrease in the circulating platelet count following an intravenous injection of heparin was first noted in mice and dogs in 1942[2] and has since been recognized as a nearly universal occurrence.[3, 4] This mild thrombocytopenia is thought to be secondary to platelet agglutination or sequestration and appears to be of trivial clinical consequence.[4-6] This mild, transient thrombocytopenia, however, must be distinguished from a severe thrombocytopenia associated with thrombosis, which can complicate heparin therapy.[6-10] This syndrome has been referred to as heparin-induced or heparin-associated thrombocytopenia (HIT or HAT) and is believed to be an immune-mediated phenomenon.[6, 7, 10-13]

With an overall morbidity and mortality of 80 per cent and 20 per cent respectively, heparin-induced thrombocytopenia has been associated with intravascular thrombosis, arterial emboli, postoperative hemorrhage, limb loss, and sudden death.[6, 8-10, 14] The purpose of this chapter is to describe the diagnostic evaluation of a patient with suspected HIT, to review the pathogenesis of this syndrome, and to outline a management approach for patients with confirmed HIT who may require further exposure to heparin.

CLINICAL PRESENTATION

Heparin-induced thrombocytopenia should be suspected in any patient who develops new thrombocytopenia (<100,000/μl), who requires increasing amounts of heparin to maintain therapeutic anticoagulation, or who demonstrates extension or de novo occurrence of a thrombotic event while receiving seemingly appropriate heparin therapy. Typically, thrombocytopenia occurs 7 to 14 days after the initiation of heparin therapy. Intravenous and subcutaneous administration of heparin as well as heparin flush have been associated with the development of HIT.[8] In addition, prior exposure to heparin seems to accelerate its appearance, and thrombocytopenia or thrombosis can occur immediately in previously sensitized patients.[7, 10, 15]

The average age of affected patients has ranged from 40 to 76 years, which most likely correlates with a need for heparinization in this age group. No difference in male/female prevalence has been noted. The nadir of the platelet count is typically 50,000/μl, although this can be quite variable.[6, 8, 10]

Once a patient develops HIT with a thombotic event, the morbidity and mortality are exceptionally high. The thrombotic complications associated with the syndrome are frequently severe and include arterial emboli or thromboses, deep venous thromboses, myocardial infarctions, cerebrovascular accidents, mesenteric infarctions, and skin infarctions.[8, 10] Management of the complications of HIT has been reported to prolong hospital stays by up to 50 days. In one series of 63 patients with HIT, 22 additional operations, including five lower extremity amputations, were required to manage the complications of heparin, and 14 deaths could be directly attributed to heparin.[10]

INCIDENCE

The exact incidence of HIT has been the subject of much debate and controversy. Earlier reports have quoted an incidence as high as 30 per cent, while later series have reported lower incidences of 0 to 5 per cent.[4-6, 10, 16-18] Much of this variability results from differing diagnostic criteria as well as from different methods of surveillance. Including all routes of heparin administration (intravenous, subcutaneous, and flush) would also alter the denominator of patients evaluated and, thus, the reported incidence.[8] To further confuse matters, the various in vitro tests used to document heparin-induced platelet activation vary considerably in sensitivity and specificity.[8, 19-21] Given these considerations, the incidence of heparin-induced platelet activation associated with thrombosis appears to be closer to 0.5 to 5 per cent of all patients receiving heparin than to the 30 per cent previously reported.[6, 10]

Several prospective studies have evaluated the relative incidence of HIT using either porcine mucosa or beef lung heparin. Although the methods of confirming the diagnosis vary, it appears that there is a higher incidence of HIT in patients who receive beef lung heparin.[5, 18, 22] Since heparin is a polydispersed compound with a molecular weight ranging from 4,000 to 20,000 daltons,[23-25] this suggests variable antigenicity with different heparin preparations. Further support for this hypothesis arises from the different reported incidences of HIT with different lots of heparin, regardless of source.[26]

The presence of a contaminant as the antigenic determinant has also been proposed but appears less likely, since the sera of patients who develop HIT will usually induce platelet activation in the presence of either beef heparin or pork heparin, regardless of which type was initially used.[8, 27, 28]

DIAGNOSIS

Since most patients receive heparin for underlying thrombotic disorders, discontinuation of heparin is not without risk and can create major problems. Thus, it is essential to establish an unequivocal diagnosis. Unfortunately, the various in vitro tests used to diagnose this syndrome vary considerably in sensitivity and specificity. The most frequently used diagnostic test is the platelet aggregation test,[6, 8, 29, 30] which is performed by mixing the patients's plasma or heat-inactivated serum with normal donor platelets and measuring the change in light transmittance in response to heparin (Fig. 8–1). An increase in light transmittance of more

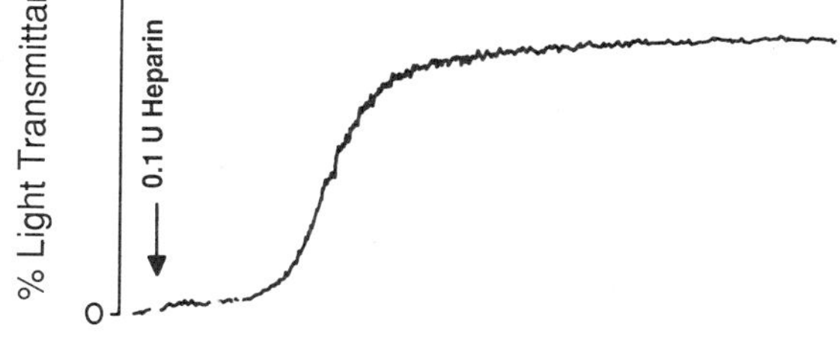

Figure 8–1. Representative in vitro platelet aggregation in response to heparin (0.1 U/ml). Baseline for 100 per cent light transmission (0 per cent absorption) is set with platelet-poor plasma. Baseline for 0 per cent light transmission (100 per cent absorption) is set with platelet-rich plasma. In response to the heparin stimulus, platelet aggregation ensues, and there is increased light transmission.

than 20 per cent within 15 to 45 minutes is considered positive.[6] In order to improve specificity, release of serotonin following platelet activation can also be measured. Furthermore, the lower the concentration of heparin required to demonstrate an effect, the more likely is the diagnosis. Thus, if the patient's plasma is mixed with normal donor platelets, and heparin (0.1 U/ml) induces 20 per cent platelet aggregation and 6 per cent serotonin release,[6, 7] the diagnosis of HIT is quite specific but somewhat insensitive. The patient's own platelets, however, are more likely than donor platelets to demonstrate a positive response.[8, 20, 31] Therefore, in order to improve the diagnostic sensitivity of this test in questionable cases, we re-evaluate the patient's own platelets following cessation of heparin therapy when the platelet count has risen.

Measurement of platelet-associated IgG has also been employed as an aide to diagnosis. Platelet-associated IgG is increased in patients with HIT.[7, 10] Unfortunately, platelet-associated IgG is elevated in other types of drug-induced thrombocytopenias, making the specificity of this test too low to be of diagnostic value.[32] The use of an enzyme-linked immunosorbent assay to measure changes in platelet-associated IgG in response to heparin may improve the diagnostic sensitivity and specificity of this assay.[33]

In summary, if HIT is suspected, platelet aggregation and serotonin release in response to heparin should be assessed. If greater than 20 per cent platelet aggregation and/or 6 per cent release of serotonin occurs, the diagnosis is confirmed. If these tests are negative or equivocal but clinical suspicion remains high, these tests should be repeated with the patient's platelets after heparin has been discontinued and the platelet count has risen. Until a diagnostic test with greater sensitivity and specificity is devised, clinical judgment continues to play an important role in establishing the diagnosis and treatment of this syndrome.

MECHANISM

Although the exact mechanisms involved in the genesis of HIT and the precise pathways required for heparin-induced platelet activation remain incompletely defined, most investigators agree that HIT is an immune-mediated phenomenon.[7, 10, 12, 13, 16] A heparin-antibody interaction was first hypothesized by Roberts et al. as a cause for recurrent arterial emboli in 1964[9]; a factor capable of aggregating platelets in the presence of heparin was subsequently identified in the plasma of a patient with HIT in 1973.[30] Since that time, this heparin-dependent platelet aggregating factor has been isolated in the IgG and IgM fractions of patients' sera.[7, 13, 16, 34] This factor has been shown to fix complement to platelet membranes,[6, 7, 12, 30] requiring an intact complement sequence to induce platelet activation.[7] The absorption of an immunoglobulin-heparin complex to platelet lysates in the presence of affected patients' sera has also been demonstrated.[13] These findings suggest that heparin acts as a hapten with an antibody directed against the heparin-platelet membrane determinant. With heparin as a co-factor, this antibody induces platelet activation in a complement-dependent, nonlytic fashion.

Despite significant progress in demonstrating that HIT is an immunological phenomenon, the biochemical pathways utilized for platelet activation are unknown. Using metabolic inhibitors and platelets from patients with either Glanzmann's thrombasthenia or Bernard-Soulier syndrome, Chong and Castaldi demonstrated that heparin-induced platelet activation requires metabolic energy and, thus, is not due to passive agglutination.[11, 12] In addition, heparin-induced aggregation requires the membrane glycoproteins IIb/IIIa, but not Ib, indicating the importance of fibrinogen in heparin-induced platelet aggregation.[11]

Further insight into the pathways involved have come from studying the effects of various platelet inhibitors on heparin-induced platelet activation. In general, depending on the strength of the stimulus, platelet activation can require thromboxane A_2 synthesis with release of endogenous ADP or can proceed by pathways independent of thromboxane A^2 synthesis or aggregation.[35-37] Thus, several investigators have demonstrated that aspirin prevents heparin-induced platelet aggregation in most patients, indicating that thromboxane A_2 synthesis is required for platelet activation in these patients.[12, 28, 38] However, other investigators have found that aspirin does not prevent heparin-induced platelet activation in all patients, indicating that other metabolic pathways may be involved.[8, 11, 28, 39-41] In this subset of patients, heparin can cause release of lysosomal hydrolases[39] and thus appears to act as a "strong" platelet agonist similar to thrombin.[35, 42, 43] Only by elevating intracellular levels of cyclic AMP (cAMP) with PGE_1 or with the prostacyclin analogue iloprost (ZK36374)[8, 11, 40, 41] (Fig. 8–2) can heparin-induced platelet activation be prevented in this subset of patients in whom heparin is acting as a strong agonist (Fig. 8–3). Whether these differing characteristics of platelet activation represent different "titers" or strengths of the heparin-dependent antibody, or completely different antibody-platelet affinities and binding characteristics, requires further investigation.

The high incidence of thrombotic as opposed to hemorrhagic complications seen in HIT distinguishes this syndrome from other drug-induced thrombocytopenias.[32] Heparin-dependent antibodies from patients with confirmed HIT have been demonstrated to bind to endothelial cells in culture and also to fix complement to these endothelial cells even in the absence of heparin.[15] This binding has been shown to damage endothelial cells and to stimulate production of tissue factor. In addition, the heparin-dependent antibodies cross-react with heparan sulfate, a naturally occur-

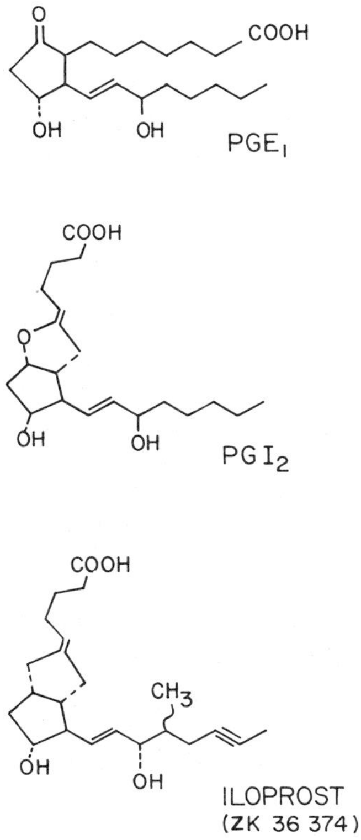

Figure 8–2. Chemical structures of the prostanoids PGE$_1$, prostacyclin (PGI$_2$), and iloprost (ZK 36374). (From Kappa JR, Fisher CA, Cottrell ED, Addonizio VP: Heparin-induced platelet activation in 16 surgical patients: Diagnosis and management. J Vasc Surg 5:101–109, 1987; and from Kappa JR, Horn MK III, Fisher CA, et al.: Efficacy of iloprost (ZK 36374) vs. aspirin in preventing heparin-induced platelet activation during open cardiac surgery. J Thorac Cardiovasc Surg 94:405–413, 1987.)

ring anticoagulant, which binds to endothelial cells.[15] Thus, immune-mediated damage of endothelial cells may alter the nature of their surface milieu, thereby increasing the procoagulant potential of the vessel wall. In conjunction with activation of circulating platelets by heparin, these endothelial changes certainly help to explain the high incidence of thrombotic complications seen in this syndrome.

MANAGEMENT

Because of the high morbidity and mortality associated with this syndrome, prevention and early diagnosis of HIT are extremely important. Daily platelet counts for patients receiving heparin have been suggested by many authors to permit early diagnosis prior to the onset of thrombotic complications.[10] However, the expense of such an approach may be prohibitive,[6] especially since thrombotic complications may occur

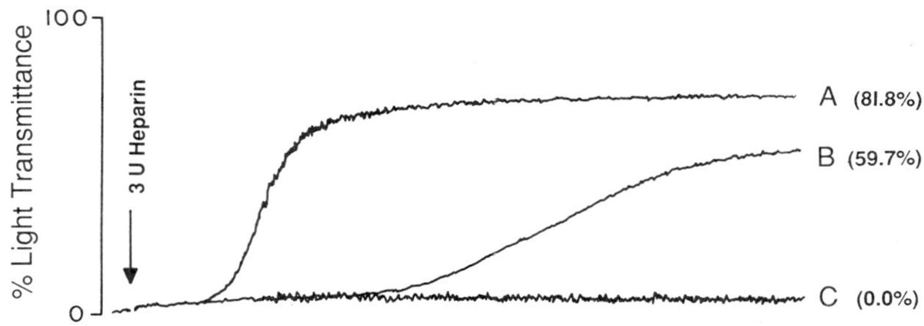

Figure 8–3. Representative in vitro platelet aggregation for a patient with HIT: with no platelet inhibitors added (A), with 40 mmol/L aspirin added (B), and with 0.01 μmol/L iloprost added to the cuvette (C). Percentages in parentheses represent the per cent ^{14}C serotonin release recorded for each aggregation curve. (From Kappa JR, Fisher CA, Cottrell ED, Addonizio VP: Heparin-induced platelet activation in 16 surgical patients: Diagnosis and management. J Vasc Surg 5:101–109, 1987; and from Kappa JR, Horn MK III, Fisher CA, et al.: Efficacy of iloprost (ZK 36374) vs. aspirin in preventing heparin-induced platelet activation during open cardiac surgery. J Thorac Cardiovasc Surg 94:405–413, 1987.)

prior to a clinical drop in the circulating platelet count.[8] Earlier institution of oral anticoagulants has also been proposed to minimize the length of exposure to heparin and thus decrease the potential for developing heparin-dependent antibodies. In addition, with earlier institution of oral agents, anticoagulation can be maintained if heparin must be discontinued.

If the diagnosis of HIT is confirmed, cessation of heparin administration is strongly advised. If continuation of antithrombotic treatment is required, other forms of anticoagulation or perhaps lytic therapy should be instituted. Since patients may be most prone to thromboses when their platelet counts are rising, oral antiplatelet agents may also prevent further thrombotic complications once heparin is discontinued.[44]

There are patients with confirmed HIT, however, for whom continued exposure or re-exposure to heparin is unavoidable. An example of these are patients requiring cardiac or vascular surgical procedures. Indeed, the thrombotic complications associated with HIT may indicate the surgical procedure. Since re-exposure to heparin can lead to intravascular activation of circulating platelets,[7, 15, 45] other clinical strategies are mandatory in these difficult management situations.

In patients requiring cardiac surgery, delay in the hope that the plasma activity of the heparin-dependent activating factor will decline has been proposed.[31] However, this approach is complicated by the variable length of time required for the factor to disappear[7, 10] and also by the unpredictable response to even one dose of heparin.[41, 46]

Since heparin is the etiological agent in this syndrome, the use of other forms of anticoagulation has also been evaluated. Low molecular weight heparins with fewer "antiplatelet properties"[25, 47] have been used successfully in certain settings.[48] These fractions presumably lack the antigenic determinants of higher molecular weight heparins and thus should not cross-react. However, these heparins have failed to prevent heparin-induced platelet activation in 20 to 40 per cent of the patients evaluated.[48, 49] The heparinoid ORG 10172 has demonstrated greater efficacy than the low molecular weight heparins in vitro[28] and has been successfully used in a patient with deep venous thrombosis.[50] However, more precise testing of the anticoagulation level provided by ORG 10172 and a means to reverse its effects are required before this approach becomes clinically feasible. A pentosaccharide composed of the precise binding sequence that mediates heparin binding to antithrombin-III is also under investigation.[51] Whether use of this compound will prevent complications now associated with heparin, including heparin-induced platelet activation, is unknown at present.

Since the majority of the complications of this syndrome are platelet-mediated, pharmacological inhibition of platelet function during heparin exposure has been used previously with variable success.[38, 40, 41, 45, 46] Aspirin inhibits platelet activation by irreversibly acetylating cyclooxygenase, thus preventing prostaglandin endoperoxide and thromboxane A_2 synthesis.[52, 53] Since heparin-induced platelet activation does not proceed by thromboxane-dependent pathways in all patients, aspirin, predictably, has a high failure rate. Janson et al. did report the successful use of aspirin to permit hemodialysis in a patient with HIT.[38] However, use of aspirin in a patient requiring cardiopulmonary bypass (CPB) did not prevent a precipitous drop in the circulating platelet count following heparin administration.[45] In addition, the effects of aspirin on platelet function are irreversible and are associated with excessive postoperative bleeding in the cardiac surgical patient.[54]

By elevation of intracellular levels of cAMP,[55] the prostanoids successfully prevent in vitro heparin-induced platelet activation even in patients in whom aspirin is not effective.[8, 11, 39-41] Iloprost (ZK36374) is a synthetic analogue of prostacyclin that was synthesized specifically as an antiplatelet agent[56, 57] (see Fig. 8–2). It is 10 times more potent than its parent compound, prostacyclin, and has fewer vasoactive side effects, which makes its clinical use technically feasible.[55] Iloprost has been used successfully to prevent heparin-induced platelet activation in nine patients undergoing urgent cardiac surgery and in one patient requiring carotid endarterectomy.[40, 41, 46]

In patients with confirmed HIT who require cardiac surgery, we begin a continuous infusion of iloprost at the induction of anesthesia. Prior to administration of heparin, plasma samples are evaluated in vitro to assess the efficacy of iloprost in inhibiting platelet function (as measured by aggregation in response to ADP), and in preventing heparin-induced platelet activation (as measured by aggregation in response to heparin) (Fig. 8–4). After ascertaining that 3 U/ml of heparin (approximately the plasma concentration achieved during bypass)[58] does not induce platelet activation in vitro, 300 U/kg heparin is administered and CPB is performed per routine. Following bypass, protamine is administered and the heparin-protamine complex is cleared via the reticuloendothelial system. At this juncture, with heparin no longer present to induce platelet activation, the iloprost infusion is discontinued. Since iloprost has a relatively short half-life, and its platelet inhibitory effects do not outlast its presence in plasma,[56] normal platelet function returns, which is clearly desirable for postoperative hemostasis. Patients treated by this protocol have had significant preservation of their platelet counts and bleeding times, despite the additive stress of synthetic surface-induced and heparin-induced platelet alterations[40, 46, 53, 59] (Figs. 8–5 and 8–6).

SUMMARY

HIT is associated with an extremely high morbidity and mortality. Careful clinical surveillance and in vitro assessment of heparin-induced

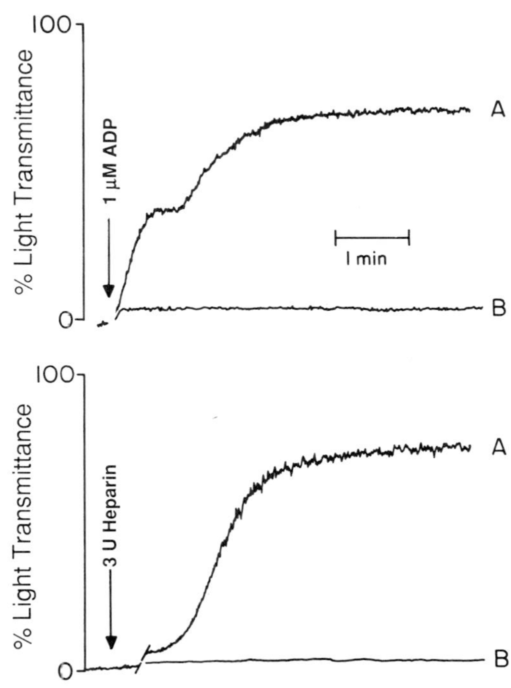

Figure 8–4. Representative platelet aggregation in response to ADP *(top)* and heparin *(bottom)* immediately after induction of anesthesia, but prior to iloprost infusion (A), and after 20 minutes of infusing iloprost at a rate of 24 ng/kg/min for a patient with HIT undergoing open-heart surgery (B).

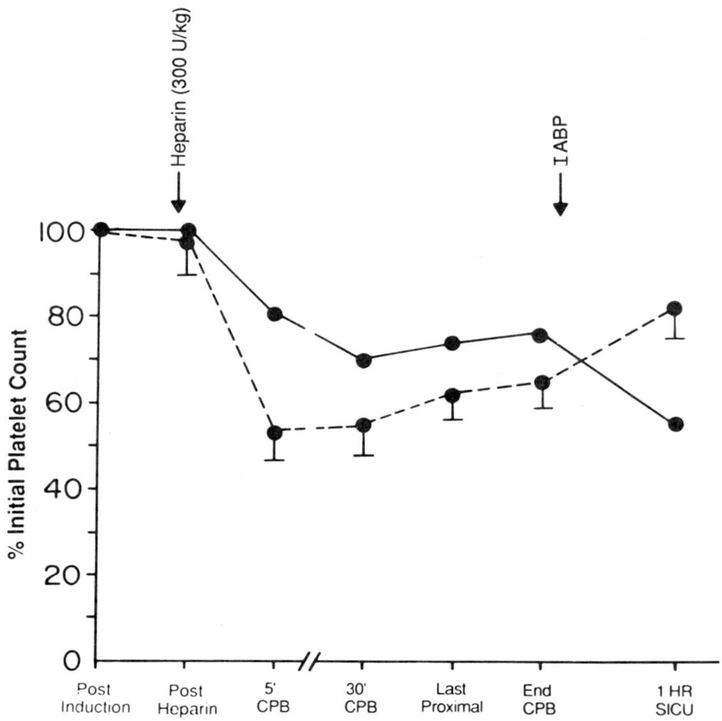

Figure 8–5. Mean whole blood platelet counts plotted against time for a patient with HIT undergoing open-heart surgery (●—●) compared with a group of historical controls (n = 21, ●- - -●) undergoing elective coronary revascularization.

platelet activation are essential for early diagnosis and reduction of associated thrombotic complications. Any patient who develops thrombocytopenia or further thrombotic complications, or in whom heparin therapy does not produce adequate anticoagulation with usual clinical doses, should be evaluated for HIT. If the diagnosis is confirmed, cessation of heparin, institution of other forms of anticoagulation, and antiplatelet therapy may reduce the complications associated with this syndrome. However, if a patient with confirmed HIT requires re-exposure to heparin, prevention of intravascular platelet activation during heparin exposure is essential. In some patients, heparin-induced platelet activation proceeds by thromboxane-dependent pathways and thus may be prevented with cyclo-oxygenase inhibitors, such as aspirin. However, in many patients, heparin-induced platelet activation proceeds by thromboxane-independent pathways. This necessitates the use of a more effective agent such as iloprost, in order to prevent the adverse sequelae of intravascular heparin-induced platelet activation.

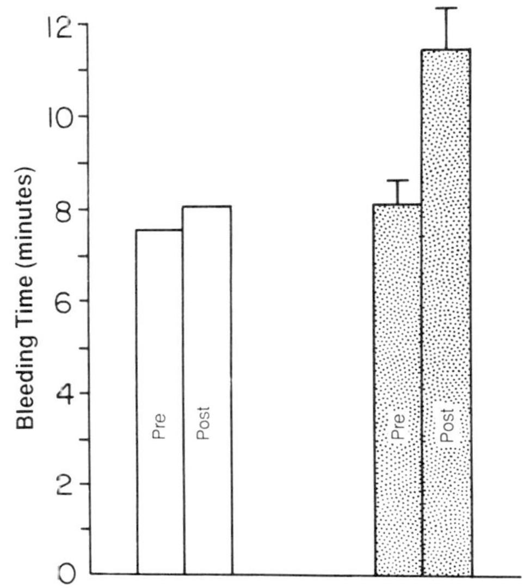

Figure 8–6. Preoperative and postoperative template bleeding times for a patient with HIT undergoing open-heart surgery (with bars) compared with a group of historical controls (n = 21, stippled bars) undergoing elective coronary revascularization. (From Kappa JR, Horn MK III, Fisher CA, et al.: Efficacy of iloprost (ZK 36374) vs. aspirin in preventing heparin-induced platelet activation during open cardiac surgery. J Thorac Cardiovasc Surg 94:405–413, 1987.)

References

1. McLean J: The thromboplastic action of cephalin. Am J Physiol 41:250–257, 1916.
2. Copley AL, Robb TB: The effect of heparin on the platelet count in dogs and mice. Am J Physiol 133:248, 1941.
3. Gollub S, Ulin AW: Heparin-induced thrombocytopenia in man. J Lab Clin Med 59:430–435, 1962.
4. Bell WR, Romasulo PA, Alving BM, Duffy TP: Thrombocytopenia occurring during the administration of heparin: A prospective study in 52 patients. Ann Intern Med 85:155–160, 1976.
5. Bell WR, Royall RM: Heparin associated thrombocytopenia: A comparison of three heparin preparations. N Engl J Med 303:902–907, 1980.
6. King DJ, Kelton JG: Heparin-associated thrombocytopenia. Ann Intern Med 100:535–540, 1984.
7. Cines DB, Kaymin P, Bina M, et al.: Heparin-associated thrombocytopenia. N Engl J Med 303:788–795, 1980.
8. Kappa JR, Fisher CA, Berkowitz HB, et al.: Heparin-induced platelet activation in sixteen surgical patients: Diagnosis and management. J Vasc Surg 5:101–109, 1987.
9. Roberts B, Rosato FE, Rosato EF: Heparin: A cause of arterial emboli? Surgery 55:803–808, 1964.
10. Silver D, Kapsch DN, Tsoi EKM: Heparin-induced thrombocytopenia, thrombosis, and hemorrhage. Ann Surg 198:301–306, 1983.
11. Chong BH, Castaldi PA: Heparin-induced thrombocytopenia: Further studies of the effects of heparin-dependent antibodies on platelets. Br J Haematol 64:347–354, 1986.
12. Chong BH, Grace CS, Rosenberg MC: Heparin-induced thrombocytopenia: Effect of heparin platelet antibody on platelets. Br J Haematol 49:531–540, 1981.
13. Green D, Harris K, Reynolds N, et al.: Heparin immune thrombocytopenia: Evidence

for a heparin-platelet complex as the antigenic determinant. J Lab Clin Med 91:167–175, 1978.
14. Weismann RE, Tobin RW: Arterial embolism occurring during systemic heparin therapy. Arch Surg 76:219–229, 1958.
15. Cines DB, Tamaski A, Tannenbaum S: Immune endothelial cell injury in heparin-associated thrombocytopenia. N Engl J Med 316:581–589, 1987.
16. Babcock RB, Dumper CW, Scharfman WB: Heparin-induced immune thrombocytopenia. N Engl J Med 295:237–241, 1976.
17. Cipolle RJ, Rodvold KA, Seifert R, et al.: Heparin-associated thrombocytopenia: A prospective evaluation of 211 patients. Ther Drug Monit 5:205–211, 1983.
18. Godal HC: Report of the International Committee on Thrombosis and Haemostasis: Thrombocytopenia and heparin. Thromb Haemost 43:222–234, 1980.
19. Kelton JG, Sheridan D, Brian H, et al.: Clinical usefulness of testing for a heparin-dependent aggregating factor in patients with suspected heparin-associated thrombocytopenia. J Lab Clin Med 103:606–612, 1984.
20. Salem HH, Van der Weyden MD: Heparin-induced thrombocytopenia. Variable platelet rich plasma reactivity to heparin dependent platelet aggregating factor. Pathology 15:297–299, 1983.
21. Sheridan D, Kelton JG: A diagnostic test for heparin-induced thrombocytopenia. Blood 67:27–30, 1986.
22. Arthur CK, Isbister JP, Aspery EM: The heparin-induced thrombosis-thrombocytopenia syndrome (H.I.T.T.S.): A review. Pathology 17:82–86, 1985.
23. Fareed J: Heparin, its fractions, fragments, and derivatives. Semin Thromb Hemost 11:1–9, 1985.
24. Messmore HL: Clinical use of heparin fractions, fragments and heparinoids. Semin Thromb Hemost 11:208–212, 1985.
25. Salzman EW, Rosenberg RD, Smith MH, et al.: Effect of heparin fractions on platelet aggregation. J Clin Invest 65:64–73, 1980.
26. Stead RB, Schafer AI, Rosenberg RD, et al.: Heterogenicity of heparin lots associated with thrombocytopenia and thromboembolism. Am J Med 77:185–188, 1985.
27. Guay DRP, Richard A: Heparin-induced thrombocytopenia—Association with a platelet aggregating factor and cross-sensitivity to bovine and porcine heparin. Drug Intell Clin Pharm 18:398–401, 1984.
28. Makhoul RG, Greenberg CS, McCann RL: Heparin-associated thrombocytopenia and thrombosis: A serious clinical problem and potential solution. J Vasc Surg 4:522–528, 1986.
29. Frantantoni JC, Pollet R, Gralnick HR: Heparin-induced thrombocytopenia: Confirmation of diagnosis with in vitro methods. Blood 45:395–401, 1975.
30. Rhodes GR, Dixon RH, Silver D: Heparin-induced thrombocytopenia with thrombotic and hemorrhagic manifestations. Surg Gynecol Obstet 136:409–416, 1973.
31. Olinger GN, Hussey CV, Olive JA, Malik MI: Cardiopulmonary bypass for patients with previously documented heparin-induced platelet aggregation. J Thorac Cardiovasc Surg 87:673–677, 1984.
32. Hackett T, Kelton JG, Powers P: Drug-induced platelet destruction. Semin Thromb Hemost 8:116–137, 1982.
33. Howe SE, Lynch DM: An enzyme-linked immunosorbent assay for the evaluation of thrombocytopenia induced by heparin. J Lab Clin Med 105:554–559, 1985.
34. Wahl TO, Lipschitz DA, Stechschulte DJ: Thrombocytopenia associated with anti-heparin antibody. JAMA 240:2560–2562, 1978.
35. Holmsen H, Day HJ: Concepts of the blood platelet release reaction. Semin Hematol 4:3–27, 1971.
36. Weiss HJ: Platelet physiology and abnormalities of platelet function, I. N Engl J Med 293:531–540, 1975.
37. Weiss HJ: Platelet physiology and abnormalities of platelet function, II. N Engl J Med 293:580–588, 1975.
38. Janson PA, Moake JL, Carpinito G: Aspirin prevents heparin-induced platelet aggregation in vivo. Br J Haematol 53:166–168, 1983.
39. Kappa JR, Fisher CA, Addonizio VP: Heparin-induced platelet activation: The role of thromboxane A_2 synthesis and the extent of platelet granule release (in preparation).

40. Kappa JR, Horn MK III, Fisher CA, et al.: Efficacy of iloprost (ZK36374) versus aspirin in preventing heparin-induced platelet activation during open cardiac surgery. J Thorac Cardiovasc Surg 94:405–413, 1987.
41. Kappa JR, Cottrell ED, Berkowitz HD, et al.: Carotid endarterectomy in patients with heparin-induced platelet activation: Comparative efficacy of aspirin and iloprost (ZK36374). J Vasc Surg 15:693–761, 1987.
42. Addonizio VP, Strauss JF, Chang LF, et al.: Release of lysosomal hydrolases during simulated extracorporeal circulation. J Thorac Cardiovasc Surg 84:28–34, 1982.
43. Holmsen H, Day HJ: The selectivity of the thrombin-induced platelet release reaction: Subcellular localization of released and retained constituents. J Lab Clin Med 75:840–855, 1970.
44. Nelson JC, Lerner RG, Goldstein R, Cagen NA: Heparin-induced thrombocytopenia. Arch Intern Med 138:548–552, 1978.
45. Smith JP, Walls JT, Muscato MS, et al.: Extracorporeal circulation in a patient with heparin-induced thrombocytopenia. Anesthesiology 62:363–365, 1985.
46. Addonizio VP, Kappa JR, Fisher CA, Ellison N: Prevention of heparin-induced thrombocytopenia during open heart surgery with ZK36374 (iloprost). Surgery 102:796–807, 1987.
47. Huisse M-G, Guillin M-C, Bezeaud A, et al.: Heparin-associated thrombocytopenia. In vitro effects of different molecular weight heparin fractions. Thromb Res 27:485–490, 1982.
48. Leroy J, Leclerc MH, DelaHousse B, et al.: Treatment of heparin associated thrombocytopenia and thrombosis with low molecular weight heparin (CY216). Semin Thromb Hemost 11:326–329, 1985.
49. Roussi JH, Houbouyan LL, Goguel AF: Use of low molecular weight heparin in heparin-induced thrombocytopenia with thrombotic complications. Lancet 1:1183, 1984.
50. Harenburg J, Zimmerman R, Schwartz F, Kubler W: Treatment of heparin-induced thrombocytopenia with thrombosis by a new heparinoid. Lancet 1:986–987, 1983.
51. Choay J: Biologic studies on chemically synthesized pentasaccharide and tetrasaccharide fragments. Semin Thromb Hemost 11:81–85, 1985.
52. Addonizio VP, Smith JB, Guiod LR, et al.: The relationship between thromboxane synthesis and platelet release during simulated extracorporeal circulation. Blood 54:371–376, 1979.
53. Roth GJ, Majerus PW: The mechanism of the effect of aspirin on human platelets. I. Acetylation of a particulate fraction protein. J Clin Invest 56:624–632, 1975.
54. Torosian M, Michelson EL, Morganroth J, McVaugh H: Aspirin and coumadin-related bleeding after coronary artery bypass graft surgery. Ann Intern Med 89:325–328, 1978.
55. Fisher CA, Kappa JR, Sinha AK, et al.: Comparison of equimolar concentrations of iloprost, prostacyclin and prostaglandin E_1 on human platelet function. J Lab Clin Med. 109:184–190, 1987.
56. Addonizio VP Jr, Fisher CA, Jenkin BK, et al.: Iloprost (ZK36374), a stable analogue of prostacyclin, preserved platelets during simulated extracorporeal circulation. J Thorac Cardovasc Surg 89:926–933, 1985.
57. Schror K, Darius H, Matzky R, Ohlendorf R: The antiplatelet and cardiovascular actions of a new carbacyclin derivative (ZK36374) equipotent to PGI_2 in vitro. Naunyn Schmiedeberg's Arch Pharmacol 316:252–255, 1981.
58. Umlas J, Jaff RH, Gauvin G, Swierk P: Anticoagulant monitoring and neutralization during open heart surgery: A rapid method for measuring heparin and calculating safe reduced protamine doses. Anesth Analg 62:1095–1099, 1983.
59. Addonizio VP, Colman RW: Platelets and extracorporeal circulation. Biomaterials 3:9–15, 1982.

CHAPTER 9

DESMOPRESSIN ACETATE IN HEMORRHAGIC CONDITIONS, WITH EMPHASIS ON USE AFTER CARDIOPULMONARY BYPASS

J. ANTHONY WARE

CAUSES OF BLEEDING FOLLOWING CARDIOPULMONARY BYPASS

Bleeding after cardiopulmonary bypass (CPB) is a serious problem that necessitates transfusion in a high percentage of patients[64] and requires the surgeon to re-explore the chest in about 3 per cent of these cardiac patients. Clinical hemorrhage has been associated with many hemostatic abnormalities produced by CPB,[7] and postoperative bleeding appears to be worse in patients with known preoperative platelet defects, such as those associated with cyanotic congenital heart disease.[77] Although most authorities recommend a battery of screening tests for the patient before CPB, including prothrombin time (PT), partial thromboplastin time (PTT), platelet count, and bleeding time,[6] the sensitivity and specificity of these measures are limited, so that prevention of bleeding by means other than using screening tests to identify those at risk is a desirable goal. The defect in hemostasis that occurs in patients during CPB has many aspects, including thrombocytopenia[79, 80] (that appears to be at least partially due to dilution),[20] impaired platelet adhesion[5] (a qualitative defect in platelet function[65, 66] that has been attributed to reduced fibrinogen receptors),[53] reduced platelet alpha$_2$-adrenergic receptors,[76] mild fibrinolysis,[75] unneutralized heparin,[22] excessive protamine,[2] and other factors. Many of these platelet abnormalities may reflect partial activation with subsequent refractoriness,[30] as is seen especially in association with certain kinds of oxygenators.[20, 67, 65] In addition, hypofibrinogenemia[56] and isolated and combined factor deficiencies[21, 79, 80] have been described.

During CPB, platelets that preoperatively aggregate to the antibiotic ristocetin become refractory to this agonist.[41] Since ristocetin-induced aggregation is dependent upon the binding of von Willebrand's factor (vWF) to a receptor on the platelet surface, this observation suggests that the vWF level may be reduced during bypass, either as a direct consequence of contact with artificial surfaces, as a result of inhibition by protamine or heparin, or by other factors. Recently, we have completed a double-blind, placebo-controlled study that demonstrated that the administration of 1-deamino-8-D-arginine vasopressin (desmopressin acetate, or DDAVP) reduces blood loss in patients undergoing certain cardiac operations.[64] Desmopressin acetate is a synthetic analogue of the antidiuretic hormone L-arginine vasopressin and has been shown to shorten the bleeding time in certain forms of hemophilia, von Willebrand's disease, uremia, and other conditions,[35, 44, 48] presumably by inducing the release of large multimers of vWF.[61] The favorable effect observed with desmopressin suggests that an abnormality of vWF occurs during CPB, is related to perioperative hemorrhage, and is corrected by desmopressin acetate. However, it must be noted that desmopressin acetate has been shown to improve hemostasis in conditions with no known abnormality of Factor VIII coagulant activity (VIII:C) or vWF.[35, 46] For the purposes of this review, Factor VIII:C will be defined as the property of normal plasma, absent in patients with hemophilia, that is measured in standard coagulation assays and is due to the presence of a procoagulant glycoprotein (Factor VIII, or antihemophiliac plasma factor) that can be identified by immunoassay. vWF is a large polymeric glycoprotein required for normal platelet adhesion and a normal bleeding time. The two are noncovalently bound and are closely associated in plasma but have different functions and different immunological properties and are the products of different genes.

CLINICAL PHARMACOLOGY OF DESMOPRESSIN ACETATE

Desmopressin acetate was first reported to increase Factor VIII:C and vWF by Cash et al.[13] and by Mannucci,[43, 45] and was also found to increase levels of tissue plasminogen activator.[25] The drug was first used for the management of bleeding problems by Mannucci et al.,[48] who gave desmopressin during dental extraction and major surgical procedures in patients with mild hemophilia and von Willebrand's disease. These investigators found that the surgical procedures could be carried out without the administration of blood products, which demonstrated that the endogenous vWF released by desmopressin was as effective as exogenously transfused factors (e.g., those in cryoprecipitate [CP]). Side effects consisted mostly of mild facial flushing, minor falls in systolic and diastolic blood pressure, and a clinically insignificant antidiuretic effect. The results of Mannucci et al. have been confirmed, and desmopressin is now an accepted part of therapy for hemophilia and many types of von Willebrand's disease. Its actions on Factor VIII:C, vWF, and tissue plasminogen activator are shared by other drugs, including nicotinic acid, insulin, adrenaline, vasopressin, and vasopressin derivatives.[42]

The pharmacokinetics of intravenous desmopressin acetate have been studied extensively, especially its effects on Factor VIII:C and vWF. An early pharmacological study in healthy volunteers given intravenous desmopressin at a dose of 0.2 μg/kg (slightly less than the dose that we use for cardiac surgery[64]) showed an average three-fold rise in Factor VIII:C activity above resting values. The peak response occurred immediately after the infusion ended.[45] The vWF levels also increased significantly, but not to the extent seen with Factor VIII:C, and appeared to peak later than did Factor VIII:C. These increases were transient but persisted above baseline for six hours and were somewhat dose-related, with a maximal effect occurring at about 0.3 to 0.4 μg/kg.[42] Studies have shown that desmopressin in repeated doses at short intervals results in lesser increases in Factor VIII:C and vWF.[44] Desmopressin acetate can also be given intranasally and subcutaneously, although markedly lower levels of Factor VIII:C and vWF are obtained via the intranasal route, and somewhat lower levels are achieved subcutaneously, but with a marked prolongation of the peak effect.[37] Administration of this drug to both normal volunteers and patients with hemophilia shortens the activated partial thromboplastin time (aPTT), even if it is not prolonged; however, the PT is unchanged.[13]

As discussed later, vWF is thought to play a crucial role in platelet-subendothelial connective tissue interaction, which is a major determinant of the bleeding time. Because of this association, the effect of desmopressin acetate on bleeding time has been studied extensively. No decrease in bleeding time could be found in most normal subjects,[45] although it does shorten in at least some normal volunteers.[35] However, desmopressin acetate reliably decreases bleeding time in a number of disorders with acquired prolongation of bleeding time.[35, 46, 78] Platelet count and platelet aggregation do not appear to be affected by this drug.[18, 64, 70]

The above-mentioned release of tissue plasminogen activator by desmopressin acetate is accompanied by an increase in the plasminogen activator inhibitor but is not accompanied by a marked increase in plasmin in the circulation. The peak level of plasminogen activator occurs at about 10 to 30 minutes after infusion of desmopressin; the half-life is about 60 minutes. The dose of desmopressin maximally effective in elevating plasminogen activator is 0.4 μg/kg, and the increases appear to correlate with Factor VIII:C and vWF levels in normal volunteers.[47] None of these studies has been validated in patients with severe atherosclerosis or thrombosis.

Very few adverse effects are reported for desmopressin acetate. Perhaps the most significant is that of tachyphylaxis, i.e., reduced response to repeated doses of desmopressin. This appears to occur especially if repeated doses are given every 12 to 24 hours for a period of some days.[16] By no means, however, does this occur in all patients.[48] Mannucci and co-investigators have reported that tachyphylaxis occurs perhaps less frequently in von Willebrand's disease than has been reported in hemophilia. However, the reduced response can also be seen in conditions with no known abnormalities of vWF, e.g., uremia.[12] If a patient should develop tachyphylaxis, a normal response can be restored by withdrawing the drug for about three to four days.[48] Also, patients who are refractory to desmopressin acetate will respond to CP with an increase in Factor VIII:C and vWF.[12] The mechanism by which tachyphylaxis responds to desmopressin acetate is unknown. It is thought that desmopressin acetate's major method for increasing levels of Factor VIII:C and vWF is by causing a brisk release of these factors from storage sites; if so, then tachyphylaxis might reflect an exhaustion of cellular stores. Alternatively, repeated doses may interfere with the release mechanism of vWF because of insensitivity of its receptor, much as the desensitization mechanism is thought to work in platelets.

Other side effects of desmopressin acetate are less problematic. There has been much concern about induction of a systemic fibrinolytic state because of the increase in tissue plasminogen activator, as noted above. However, to date, no significant instances of such an occurrence have been reported. Unlike natural antidiurectic hormones, desmopressin has very little effect on the V_1 vasopressin receptors on smooth muscle cells and thus produces no vasoconstriction, hypertension, or contractions of visceral smooth muscle.[60]

The most common side effect seen following desmopressin acetate administration has been mild vasodilation. This manifests as facial flushing, as mild, clinically insignificant drops in systolic blood pressure, or as a 10 to 20 per cent increase in heart rate. These effects are transient and produce no problem in most anesthetized patients. Although desmopressin acetate has a potent antidiuretic effect, no cases of severe water intoxication have been associated with its use.[42]

IMPORTANCE OF vWF IN HEMOSTASIS

Since the initial description of von Willebrand's disease in 1924,[34] the importance of vWF in normal hemostasis has been increasingly appreciated. vWF appears to be a multimeric complex of macromolecules of very high molecular weight; each glycoprotein subunit has a molecular weight of about 230,000 daltons.[29] These molecules are composed of identical subunits that are connected and have multiple binding sites, features that make vWF an ideal bridging molecule.[16] Endothelial cells are presumed to be the major source of plasma vWF, although it should be noted that megakaryocytes also synthesize the macromolecule.[32, 55] vWF is also detectable in the subendothelium in vivo;[58] that which is synthesized by megakaryocytes is localized in the platelet alpha granules.[54] Platelet-associated vWF is released upon stimulation in a process that causes it to become exposed on the platelet surface.[26] Most evidence suggests that vWF's major role is to serve as a bridge for the adhesion of platelets to the subendothelium[16] or between platelets. Once vWF is expressed on the subendothelium, the platelets adhere to the immobilized form of the factor. It is also known that vWF is involved in platelet-to-platelet interactions,[73] and ADP and thrombin—both common platelet agonists—can induce the binding of vWF to platelets,[23, 24] primarily to the glycoprotein IIB/IIIA complex.[28] Thus, one might expect that a drug such as desmopressin, which increases vWF levels through release from storage sites, would have a salutory effect on hemostasis owing primarily to a promotion of platelet-to-platelet and possibly platelet-to-subendothelium interaction.

The exact mechanism by which desmopressin acetate causes an abrupt increase in Factor VIII:C activity and vWF levels is still a matter of speculation. Because of the rapidity of this response, it appears that increased synthesis cannot account for the change in levels. Also, it seems unlikely that desmopressin acetate increases the concentration of vWF by prolonging the half-life, because the autologous vWF that is increased with desmopressin acetate has a shorter half-life than the exogenous vWF that is infused in CP.[37, 44] How desmopressin acetate might cause such a release of vWF from endothelial cells is unknown. It does not appear to be a direct or local effect, since the administration of desmopressin to cultured endothelial cells in vitro or to a direct perfusate of isolated human vessels does not cause release of Factor VIII:C or vWF.[4, 52, 74] The observation that hemophiliacs with high levels of vWF after treatment with CP did not increase vWF in response to subsequent desmopressin to the extent that was seen in the same patients studied at a time when they had lower resting values of vWF[74] suggests that a systemically mediated negative feedback loop may exist for desmopressin-induced increases in vWF.

DESMOPRESSIN IN HEMOPHILIA AND VON WILLEBRAND'S DISEASE

Although desmopressin acetate has been used in many clinical situations, the first and still most widely accepted use of this drug is in patients with known abnormalities in Factor VIII:C or vWF. Considerable experience exists for the use of this drug for mild to moderate hemophilia, reported initially by Mannucci et al. [48] These clinical studies in general emphasize desmopressin's usefulness in treating acute bleeding episodes and in preventing bleeding during dental extractions or major surgical operations. The drug usually increases Factor VIII:C activity about three or four times over the resting level; however, the peak level is quite variable, and some patients have minimal or no responses, especially if they have no Factor VIII:C to begin with.[19, 42] The hemostatic effect of desmopressin acetate appears to be closely related to the level of Factor VIII:C, and the time of peak effect appears to occur soon after the infusion ends (30 to 90 minutes).[19] Several studies have also sought the proper dose of the drug and method of infusion. Most investigators have infused the drug over 15 to 30 minutes; longer infusions do not appear to increase effectiveness, but facial flushing and other manifestations of vasodilation may be decreased with longer infusions. The dose given has varied from 0.3 to 0.5 μg/kg. Higher doses do not increase Factor VIII:C activity more than is seen with 0.3 μg/kg, and thus are probably not indicated.[51]

As one might expect, desmopressin acetate has also received much attention in the treatment of patients with von Willebrand's disease. It can be used to raise the level of Factor VIII:C in a greater percentage of these patients than in those with classic hemophilia, because fewer of the patients with von Willebrand's disease have a severe form of the disease that is unresponsive to desmopressin. The prolonged bleeding time, which is one of the hallmarks of von Willebrand's disease, may not be totally corrected by desmopressin acetate, but the desired clinical effect of prevention or termination of bleeding occurs nonetheless. As with hemophilia, the correction of the Factor VIII:C defect in von Willebrand's disease appears to be more important than correction of the bleeding time to prevent postsurgical hemorrhage or spontaneous soft tissue bleeding; the bleeding time may be more closely related to mucosal hemorrhages.[8, 38]

The clinical efficacy of desmopressin acetate varies considerably among the different types of von Willebrand's disease. The most frequent form of this disease is type I, which is characterized by low plasma levels of vWF with an intact multimeric structure. Desmopressin acetate will reliably increase Factor VIII:C and provide good hemostasis in those with mild to moderate type I von Willebrand's disease, but the bleeding time may improve minimally, even in those with excellent hemostasis during surgery and normal wound healing.[19] The magnitude of responses of Factor VIII:C is about the same as that seen in hemophiliacs.[42] Patients with type II von Willebrand's disease, which is characterized by dysfunctional vWF with abnormal multimeric structure, will also have satisfactory Factor VIII:C responses to desmopressin, but in only a few subtypes will the bleeding time normalize. Special mention should be made of the subtype IIB, in which desmopressin does not shorten the prolonged bleeding time but actually causes platelet aggregation in vivo.[31] In patients with this subtype, the administration of desmopressin acetate is contraindicated. Although the subtype gives some indication as to the anticipated effect, it should be noted that for practical purposes it is very difficult to predict the response of a given individual to desmopressin.[16]

DESMOPRESSIN IN CONDITIONS WITH NO APPARENT ABNORMALITY OF FACTOR VIII:C OR vWF

Perhaps surprisingly, it has recently become clear that many acquired hemorrhagic conditions not associated with abnormalities in Factor VIII:C or vWF can be ameliorated by the use of desmopressin acetate. The most firmly established indication for desmopressin acetate in acquired bleeding disorders is uremia, because of the clear demonstration by Mannucci et al. and others[46, 78] that the bleeding time can be dramatically shortened by desmopressin, and hemorrhages following surgical procedures can be remarkably lessened or stopped with such therapy. The initial use of the drug for this condition was prompted by observations[33] that the infusion of CP could allow the safe performance of many surgical procedures. In two studies in which desmopressin acetate (0.3 or 0.4 μg/kg) was given to patients with chronic renal failure, it was noted that previously prolonged bleeding times became normal in 75 per cent of these patients, and remained normal for about 2 to 4 hours in 60 per cent of the patients, returning to the prolonged baseline state by between 8 and 24 hours. Factor VIII:C activity, which is not abnormally decreased in uremic patients, was nevertheless increased two-fold after desmopressin administration; but the platelet count, PT, and platelet cyclic AMP (cAMP) levels were not affected.[46] Although the mechanism for improvement with desmopressin is not certain, shortening of the bleeding time is temporally associated with the appearance in plasma of the higher molecular weight multimeric forms. The clinical improvement in hemostasis has permitted biopsies or major surgical operations in several subsequent studies. Thus, it appears that desmopressin allows short-term control of uremic hemorrhagic tendency without the hazards inherent in transfusion of CP; it has been suggested that desmopressin is the first choice for prevention and treatment of bleeding complications in uremic patients.[42]

There are other clinical conditions in which desmopressin acetate has been shown to prevent or reverse bleeding complications following surgical procedures. Desmopressin acetate markedly decreases the bleeding time in patients with storage pool deficiency, a congenital platelet defect associated with prolonged bleeding time and mucosal hemorrhages, and also reverses the aspirin-induced prolongation of bleeding time in normal subjects.[35] Other investigators were unable to confirm that desmopressin acetate decreases the bleeding time in patients with storage pool deficiency or with Glanzmann's thrombasthenia but did find that the drug shortens the bleeding time in patients with hepatic cirrhosis.[49] This decrease in bleeding time appears to correlate with improvement in clinical hemostasis; Kobrinsky and colleagues found that major surgery could be performed without blood product support in nine patients and minor surgery in five patients, all with prolonged bleeding times, after receiving desmopressin acetate.[35]

Furthermore, some investigations have shown that desmopressin acetate improves hemostasis in conditions in which there is not only no known abnormality or reduced level of vWF but also no prolongation of bleeding time. Such an example is reported by Kobrinsky et al.,[36] who conducted a randomized, double-blind, placebo-controlled study to evaluate the effect of desmopressin acetate on intraoperative blood loss in hemostatically normal subjects undergoing spinal fusion surgery. The patients were tested with 0.3 μg/kg of desmopressin intravenously three days before surgery. If the bleeding time was decreased, or if an increase in Factor VIII:C occurred following administration of the drug, desmopressin or placebo was administered at the time of surgery, and blood loss was compared. In their study of 16 patients, desmopressin acetate decreased operative blood loss (1080 ± 750 ml in the placebo group vs. 770 ± 500 ml in the treated group), which was predicted by the baseline effect of desmopressin on the bleeding time and Factor VIII:C level. These authors concluded that desmopressin acetate is clinically useful in the prevention of surgical blood loss, even in subjects who were hemostatically competent preoperatively.[36]

Experimental support for the concept that there is a salutary effect of desmopressin acetate on hemostasis, even in conditions with no known abnormality in vWF, was recently provided by Buchanan et al.,[10] who found that desmopressin prevented the bleeding associated with excessive heparin without inhibiting its antithrombotic effect. These authors hypothesized that desmopressin's beneficial effect was due to the reversal of heparin-induced platelet inhibition. However, vWF or its multimers were not measured in this study, so the relation between the presumed increase in vWF and the prevention of bleeding is unclear.

Much speculation has arisen as to why desmopressin acetate should improve hemostasis and/or shorten the bleeding time in clinical conditions in which no defects or abnormalities in Factor VIII:C or vWF have been identified. That at least a minimum number of platelets is required in order for desmopressin acetate to exert its beneficial effect was shown by Mannucci et al. in a study in which they found poor efficacy of the drug when given to patients with severe thrombocytopenia.[49] Some investigators have hypothesized that the drug may inhibit the generation of vascular PGI_2, because of experiments finding that human vessel segments incubated with desmopressin in vitro form lower concentrations of prostacycline metabolites in response to stimuli; the plasma levels in vivo of similar metabolites were reduced following desmopressin therapy.[9, 69] However, as mentioned above, the drug is effective in reducing bleeding time in patients treated with aspirin in doses sufficient to abolish the production of vascular prostacycline.[35] One possibility is that vWF multimers that are larger than normal are transiently released by desmopressin and might promote platelet adhesion or platelet-to-platelet interaction.[63] However, if such a mechanism were the only source of desmopressin's benefit in these conditions, then one would expect the bleeding time to be invariably shortened, which, as reviewed above, it is not. Thus, other factors must be involved. Some experimental evidence has been presented to suggest that desmopressin acts to enhance platelet adhesion onto a damaged vessel wall via a vWF-independent mechanism.[4] As noted above, this direct effect has not yet been reproduced in cell culture systems and must be regarded as speculative pending further studies.

DESMOPRESSIN FOLLOWING CARDIOPULMONARY BYPASS

It appears that desmopressin acetate may influence hemostasis both by increasing concentrations of vWF, especially the larger multimers, and by a mechanism that appears to work largely through a nonspecific enhancement of platelet function, which is possibly independent of vWF. Both of these mechanisms are pertinent to desmopressin's improvement of hemostasis following cardiac surgery. We recently completed a prospective trial determining the effect of desmopressin on operative and postoperative hemostasis in patients undergoing cardiopulmonary bypass (CPB).[64] This trial was randomized and double-blind and involved 70 patients undergoing heart operations, including valve replacement, closure of atrial septal defects, resection of ventricular aneurysm, and repeat coronary artery bypass grafting (CABG) using either the saphenous vein or internal mammary artery. Patients undergoing primary uncomplicated CABG were not included in this study because of concern that desmopressin acetate, by raising the plasma level of vWF, might create a prothrombotic state. It should be mentioned that no patient with such a state has ever been described, and that no thrombotic complications with the use of desmopressin acetate have been reported. In our study, patients were given 0.3 μg/kg of desmopressin acetate or an identical-appearing placebo after the completion of bypass, and immediately after the administration of protamine to reverse heparin. (This time was chosen so as to allow testing for a possible protamine-desmopressin interaction in effect on vWF; such an interaction was not observed). The total blood loss of the operation and in the first 24 hours was 2210 ± 1415 ml in the control group and 1317 ± 486 ml in the patients who received desmopressin acetate ($p = 0.001$). The patients receiving desmopressin acetate had less blood loss in the operating room, in the first 12 hours after operation, and in the 12th to the 24th hour after operation. One patient required recannulation and reinstitution of bypass because of hemorrhage, and two required a return to the operating room for control of bleeding. All these patients had received the placebo. Fourteen patients lost more than 2 liters of blood during operation and in the first 24 hours postoperatively; 11 of these patients received the placebo.[64]

There were no side effects of desmopressin acetate noted in our trial, and the antidiuretic effect did not appear to be important in our study, which is consistent with the previous literature. There were no differences between the control and treatment groups in terms of mean arterial pressure, urine output, weight gain, postoperative bleeding time (mean: 7.58 vs. 7.38 min), fibrinopeptide A levels, or platelet count (either preoperatively or after bypass), although the patients with desmopressin acetate tended to have more platelets postoperatively than did the placebo group (116,639 platelets/ml vs. 95,760 ± 35,920, $p = 0.04$).

Two patients died early postoperatively, one in each group. One patient in each group had a perioperative myocardial infarction. Two patients in the desmopressin group and one in the placebo group had early postoperative strokes, none of which had permanent neurological sequelae.

In a study with a different design, Czer and colleagues administered desmopressin acetate in a fixed dose of 20 μg to 23 patients with mediastinal hemorrhage and prolonged bleeding time after cardiac surgery, including 17 patients undergoing primary CABG.[17] These 17 patients were compared with 16 untreated patients who also had mediastinal hemorrhage and prolonged bleeding time and who were matched in procedure and pump time. In the treatment group, the bleeding time was corrected from 17 minutes (before desmopressin) to 12.5 minutes (after desmopressin), and the Factor VIII levels were much higher following the drug; the platelet counts were not significantly different. These authors also found that desmopressin acetate lowered subsequent blood product usage in the treatment group as compared with the control group and also significantly decreased the number of patients who underwent reoperation.

In an effort to understand the mechanism behind the beneficial effects seen with desmopressin acetate following CPB, we have performed detailed analyses of the vWF antigen concentration and activity before, during, and after bypass. In our study, the vWF antigen was quantified by electroimmunoassay according to the Laurell method.[82] Radioimmunoassay (RIA) or immunoradiometric assay (IRMA) may also be reliably used for these determinations. The electroimmunoassay employed by us is easier, and perhaps more reproducible, but is less sensitive than RIA or IRMA. vWF activity was measured by the ristocetin platelet agglutination assay. The multimers were analyzed by agarose gel electrophoresis, which requires electrophoresis of plasma through SDS agarose and identification of multimeric forms by overlaying the gel with radiolabeled antibody to vWF.[82] Multimers were quantified by densitometric measurement, and high molecular weight multimers were arbitrarily defined as those with a molecular weight greater than multimers at the densitometric curve maximum of normal pooled plasma.

Before the operation, the patients destined to be treated with desmopressin had vWF levels (in units per ml) of 1.85 $\pm$ 0.76 vs. 1.79 $\pm$ 0.78 in the placebo group, a difference that is not statistically significant. Following the drug or placebo, the patients treated with vWF had a mean level of 1.80, whereas the level had decreased during bypass to 1.46 in the group receiving placebo, a significant difference ($p < 0.02$).

An unexpected finding was a correlation of the preoperative plasma levels of vWF with the subsequent blood loss (Fig. 9–1). Patients with major bleeding tended to have the lowest preoperative vWF levels. As expected, the postoperative level of vWF was higher in patients who received desmopressin acetate than in those who received the placebo, particularly among those who had a low level of vWF before the operation. Thus, if patients with a relatively low preoperative level of vWF were at a hemostatic disadvantage, this appears to have been offset by the receipt of desmopressin acetate.

Preoperatively, patients with valvular heart disease, especially aortic stenosis, had a lower percentage of high molecular weight multimers than did those patients with coronary artery disease (61 $\pm$ 16 per cent vs. 91 $\pm$ 20 per cent, $p < 0.001$). The percentage of high molecular weight multimers in the coronary artery disease group was similar to that of healthy controls.[81] This reduction in high molecular weight multimers in the patients with valvular disease was not reflected in the bleeding time or in the ability of the platelets to aggregate to ristocetin. As noted above, the mean level of vWF had decreased by the end of bypass to about 1.3 U/ml. However, we found that the high molecular

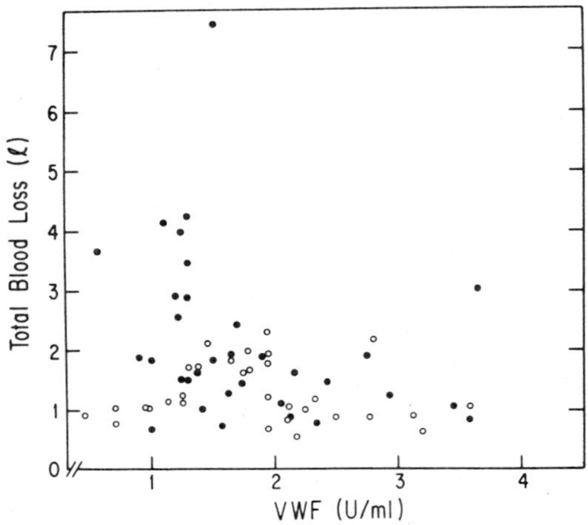

Figure 9–1. Influence of preoperative levels of von Willebrand Factor (vWF) on total blood loss for the first 24 hours postoperatively. Patients in the placebo groups are shown as open circles, and those given desmopressin acetate are shown as filled circles. (From Salzman EW, Weinstein MJ, Weintraub RM, et al.: Treatment with desmopressin acetate to reduce blood loss after cardiac surgery. N Engl J Med 314:1402–1406, 1986, by permission of the Massachusetts Medical Society.)

weight multimers increased to a similar amount in patient groups with valvular heart disease and coronary artery disease. The high molecular weight multimers increased regardless of whether the patients received desmopressin or placebo, and did not appear to differ between the patient groups with coronary artery disease or valvular heart disease. Twenty-four hours postoperatively, the mean percentage of high molecular weight multimers declined from 120 per cent of the normal value to a level that was nearly normal, and the vWF levels rose to 2.4 U/ml in both the drug and the placebo groups. We hypothesize that the vWF concentration during bypass was reduced owing to hemodilution but increased immediately postoperatively owing to its release from a storage pool as a generalized "acute phase" reaction. We were unable to correlate the increased percentage of high molecular weight forms with reduced blood loss; the vWF concentration may be a more accurate determinant. Other relevant factors that may influence the level of vWF in cardiac patients have recently been described.[1, 50] One of these studies[50] followed the course of vWF during myocardial infarction and unstable angina and found that there was no significant elevation of vWF in the blood of patients with unstable angina. However, a few days following acute myocardial infarction, the level of vWF became elevated and remained abnormal for up to 14 days. There was no evidence that vWF was released from the area of damaged myocardium itself, although the assay used in this particular study was not sensitive enough to actually disprove this hypothesis. It seems more likely that the elevation of vWF again resulted from its role as an acute phase reactant. Epidemiological studies[1] have found that elderly patients, who as a group have increased plasma concentrations of tissue plasminogen activator, also have higher levels of plasminogen activator inhibitor, which is increased in parallel with Factor VIII:C and vWF.

CURRENT AND FUTURE USES IN CARDIAC SURGICAL PATIENTS

Several questions regarding the efficacy and appropriateness of the use of desmopressin acetate in cardiac surgery remain unanswered. Although it has now been established that desmopressin acetate reduces the blood loss in patients undergoing more complex cardiac operations, the usefulness of desmopressin acetate in patients undergoing primary uncomplicated CABG was not directly tested in our study (although it has been evaluated in an unblinded fashion[17]). Since approximately 65 per cent of the cardiac operations performed in the United States are of this type, extension of the results of our study to primary CABG patients might have an important effect on national requirements for homologous blood.

Another question that has not been addressed is the ability of desmopressin acetate to reduce bleeding due to aspirin ingestion before undergoing CABG. It is now accepted practice in most centers to administer aspirin and dipyridimole to prevent early saphenous vein bypass graft closure following surgery.[14, 15, 68] However, most investigators do not recommend aspirin preoperatively, for fear that bleeding would increase.[71] It is conceivable that there might be some benefit from earlier treatment with aspirin, and, if the bleeding complications could be minimized through administration of another agent, the benefit-to-risk ratio could increase considerably. Furthermore, aspirin is commonly given before percutaneous transluminal coronary angioplasty, in the hope of preventing restenosis.[59] Occasionally, patients undergoing percutaneous transluminal coronary angioplasty will require emergent surgery; although it has not been studied directly, they might be at higher risk for intraoperative and postoperative bleeding than similar patients who do not receive aspirin or dipyridimole. In addition, two large, well-designed, placebo-controlled studies have found striking benefit from the use of aspirin for unstable angina.[11, 40] However, these patients often are referred for aortocoronary bypass surgery if medical therapy fails, and again may have increased risk of bleeding due to pretreatment with platelet-inhibiting agents. Therefore, desmopressin's ability to reverse the aspirin-induced platelet defect[35] might be important. However, the clinical implication of this effect, i.e., desmopressin-induced decrease in surgical bleeding, has not been examined.

To summarize our current practice, we recommend use of desmopressin in all complicated cardiac surgical cases in which more than minimal blood loss is expected. We do not give it to patients undergoing routine CABG unless excessive bleeding is anticipated. We also recommend the use of desmopressin in noncardiac surgical patients in whom problem bleeding develops, especially in patients whose history suggests the possibility of a drug-induced qualitative defect of platelet function, such as after aspirin ingestion. Although we believe that the data are convincing, and that our practice is founded on sound scientific principles in the type of cardiac surgical patients mentioned above, we believe that the use of desmopressin acetate in other types of cardiac surgery is unproven, although rational, and further studies will be required to determine the eventual role of this drug in cardiovascular and surgical practice.

References

1. Aillaud MF, Pignol F, Alessi MC, et al.: Increase in plasma concentration of plasminogen activator inhibitor, fibrinogen, von Willebrand factor, factor VIII:C and in erythrocyte sedimentation rate with age. Thromb Haemost 55:330–332, 1986.
2. Andersen MN, Mendelow M, Alfano GA: Experimental studies of heparin and protamine activity with special reference to protamine inhibition of clotting. Surgery 46:1060–1068, 1959.
3. Bachmann F, McKenna R, Cole ER, Najafi H: The hemostatic mechanism after open-heart surgery. I. Studies on plasma coagulation factors and fibrinolysis in 512 patients after extracorporeal circulation. J Thorac Cardiovasc Surg 70:76–85, 1975.
4. Barnhart MI, Chen S, Lusher JM: DDAVP: Does the drug have a direct effect on the vessel wall? Thromb Res 31:239–253, 1983.
5. Bhargava M, Sanyal SK, Thapar MK, et al.: Impairment of platelet adhesiveness and platelet factor 3 activity in cyanotic congenital heart disease. Acta Haematol 5:216–223, 1976.
6. Bick RL: Alterations of hemostasis associated with cardiopulmonary bypass. Semin Thromb Hemost 3:59–82, 1976.
7. Bick RL: Hemostasis defects associated with cardiac surgery, prosthetic devices and other extracorporeal circuits. Semin Thromb Hemost 11:249–280, 1985.
8. Biggs R, Matthews JM: The treatment of haemorrhage in von Willebrand's disease and the blood level of factor VIII (AHG). Br J Haematol 9:203–214, 1963.
9. Blajchmann MA, Sengi AF, Hirsh J, et al.: Shortening of the bleeding time in rabbits by hydrocortisone caused in inhibition of prostacyclin generation by the vessel wall. J Clin Invest 63:1026–1035, 1979.
10. Buchanan MR, N'guyen P, McKenna JVR, et al.: DDAVP reduces the platelet defect associated with heparin (abstract). Circulation (Suppl) 74:III–380, 1986.
11. Cairns J, Gent M, Singer J, et al.: Aspirin, sulfinpyrazone, or both in unstable angina. N Engl J Med 313:1369–1375, 1985.
12. Canavese C, Salomone M, Pacitti A, et al.: Reduced response of uraemic bleeding time to repeated doses of desmopressin. Lancet 1:867–868, 1985.
13. Cash JD, Gader AMA, DaCosta J: The release of plasminogen activator and factor VIII by LVP, AVP, DDAVP, AT III, and OT in man. Br J Haematol 27:363–364, 1974.
14. Chesebro JH, Fuster V, Elveback LR, et al.: Effect of dipyridamole and aspirin on late vein-graft patency after coronary bypass operations. N Engl J Med 310:209–214, 1984.

15. Chesebro JH, Lam JYT, Fuster V: The pathogenesis and prevention of aortocoronary vein bypass graft occlusion and restenosis after arterial angioplasty: Role of vascular injury and platelet thrombus deposition. JACC 8:57B–66B, 1986.
16. Coller BS: Von Willebrand's disease. In Ratnoff OD, Forbes CD (eds): Disorders of Hemostasis, Orlando, Grune & Stratton, 1984, pp. 241–269.
17. Czer L, Bateman T, Gray R, et al.: Prospective trial of DDAVP in treatment of severe platelet dysfunction and hemorrhage after cardiopulmonary bypass (abstract). Circulation (Suppl) 72:111–130, 1985.
18. D'Angelo A, Capitanio A, Smith JB, et al.: Effect of desamino-D-arginine vasopressin (DDAVP) on plasma levels of platelet and endothelial cell release products. Thromb Haemost 49:64–65, 1983.
19. De La Fuente B, Kasper CK, Rickles FR, Hoyer LW: Response of patients with mild and moderate hemophilia A and von Willebrand disease to treatment with desmopressin. Ann Intern Med 103:6–14, 1985.
20. Edmunds LH Jr, Ellison N, Colman RW, et al.: Platelet function during cardiac operation; comparison of membrane and bubble oxygenators. J Thorac Cardiovasc Surg 83:805–812, 1982.
21. Ekert H, Dowling SV: Platelet release abnormality and reduced prothrombin levels in children with cyanotic congenital heart disease. Aust Paediatr J 13:17–21, 1977.
22. Ellison N, Beatty CP, Blake DR, et al.: Heparin rebound: Studies in patients and volunteers. J Thorac Cardiovasc Surg 67:723–729, 1974.
23. Fujimoto T, Hawiger J: Adenosine diphosphate induces binding of von Willebrand factor to human platelets. Nature 297:154–156, 1982.
24. Fujimoto T, Ohara S, Hawiger J: Thrombin-induced exposure and prostacyclin inhibition of the receptor for factor VIII/von Willebrand factor on human platelets. J Clin Invest 69:1212–1222, 1982.
25. Gader AMA, daCosta J, Cash JD: A new vasopressin analogue and fibrinolysis. Lancet 2:1417–1418, 1973.
26. George JN, Onofre AR: Human platelet surface binding of endogenous secreted factor VIII, von Willebrand factor and platelet factor 4. Blood 59:194–197, 1982.
27. Gill JC, Wilson AD, Endres-Brooks J, Montgomery RR: Loss of the largest von Willebrand factor multimers from the plasma of patients with congenital cardiac defects. Blood 67:758–761, 1986.
28. Gralnick HR, Coller BS: Platelets stimulated with thrombin and ADP bind von Willebrand factor to different sites than platelets stimulated with ristocetin (abstract). Clin Res 31:482A, 1983.
29. Gralnick HR, Coller BS, Shulman NR, et al.: Factor VIII. Ann Intern Med 86:598–616, 1977.
30. Harker LA, Malpass TW, Branson HE, et al.: Mechanism of abnormal bleeding in patients undergoing cardiopulmonary bypass; acquired transient platelet dysfunction associated with selective α-granule release. Blood 56:824–834, 1980.
31. Holmberg L, Nilsson IM, Borge L, et al.: Platelet aggregation induced by 1-deamino-8-D-arginine vasopressin (DDAVP) in type IIB von Willebrand's disease. N Engl J Med 309:816–821, 1983.
32. Jaffe EA, Hoyer LW, Nachman RL: Synthesis of antihemophilic factor antigen by cultured human endothelial cells. J Clin Invest 52:2757–2764, 1973.
33. Janson PA, Jubelirer SJ, Weinstein MS, Deykin D: Treatment of bleeding tendency in uremia with cryoprecipitate. N Engl J Med 303:1318–1322, 1980.
34. Jorpes EJ: E.A. von Willebrand och von Willebrands sjukdom. Nord Med 67:729–732, 1962.
35. Kobrinsky NL, Israels ED, Gerrard JM, et al.: Shortening of bleeding time by 1-deamino-8-D-arginine vasopressin in various bleeding disorders. Lancet 1:1145–1148, 1984.
36. Kobrinsky NL, Israels ED, Letts M, et al.: DDAVP shortens the bleeding time and decreases operative blood loss in hemostatically normal subjects undergoing spinal-fusion surgery (abstract). Blood 66:323a, 1985.
37. Kohler M, Hellstern P, Miyashita C, et al.: Comparative study of intranasal, subcutaneous, and intravenous administration of DDAVP. Thromb Haemost 55:108–111, 1986.

38. Larrieu MJ, Caen JP, Meyer D, et al.: Congenital bleeding disorders with long bleeding time and normal platelet count. II. von Willebrand disease (report of thirty-seven patients). Am J Med 45:354–372, 1968.
39. Larrieu MJ, Soulier JP: Deficit en facteur antihemophilique A chez une fille, associé à un trouble du saignement. Rev Hematol 8:361–370, 1953.
40. Lewis HD, Davis JW, Archibald DG, et al.: Protective effects of aspirin against acute myocardial infarction and death in men with unstable angina. N Engl J Med 309:396–403, 1983.
41. Mammen EF, Koets MH, Washington BC, et al.: Hemostasis changes during cardiopulmonary bypass surgery. Semin Thromb Hemost 11:281–292, 1985.
42. Mannucci PM: Desmopressin (DDAVP) for treatment of disorders of hemostasis. In Coller BS (ed): Progress in Hemostasis and Thrombosis. Orlando, Grune & Stratton, 1986, pp 19–45.
43. Mannucci PM, Aberg M, Nilsson IM, Robertson B.: Mechanism of plasminogen activator and factor VIII increase after vasoactive drugs. Br J Haematol 30:81–93, 1975.
44. Mannucci PM, Canciani MT, Rota L, Donovan BS: Response of factor VIII/von Willebrand factor to DDAVP in healthy subjects and patients with haemophilia A and von Willebrand's disease. Br J Haematol 47:283–293, 1981.
45. Mannucci PM, Pareti FI, Holmberg L, et al.: Studies on the prolonged bleeding time in von Willebrand disease. J Lab Clin Med 88:662–671, 1976.
46. Mannucci PM, Remuzzi G, Pusineri F, et al.: Deamino-8-D-arginine vasopressin shortens the bleeding time in uremia. N Engl J Med 308:8–12, 1983.
47. Mannucci PM, Rota L: Plasminogen activator response after DDAVP: A clinico-pharmacological study. Thromb Res 20:69–76, 1980.
48. Mannucci PM, Ruggeri ZM, Pareti FI, Capitanio A: 1-Deamino-8-D-arginine vasopressin: A new pharmacological approach to the management of haemophilia and von Willebrand's disease. Lancet 1:869–872, 1977.
49. Mannucci PM, Vicente V, Vianello L, et al.: Controlled trial of desmopressin (DDAVP) in liver cirrhosis and other conditions associated with a prolonged bleeding time. Blood 67:1148–1153, 1986.
50. Margulis T, David M, Maor N, et al.: The von Willebrand factor in myocardial infarction and unstable angina: A kinetic study. Thromb Haemost 55:366–368, 1986.
51. Mariani G, Ciavarella N, Mazzucconi MG, et al.: Evaluation of the effectiveness of DDAVP in surgery and in bleeding episodes in hemophilia and von Willebrand's disease: A study of 43 patients. Clin Lab Haematol 6:229–238, 1984.
52. Moffat EH, Giddings JC, Bloom AL: The effect of deamino-D-arginine vasopressin (DDAVP) and naloxone infusion of factor VIII and possible endothelial cell related activities. Br J Haematol 57:651–662, 1984.
53. Musial J, Niewiarowski S, Hershock D, et al.: Loss of fibrinogen receptors from the platelet surface during simulated extracorporeal circulation. J Lab Clin Med 105:514–522, 1985.
54. Nachman RL, Jaffe EA: Subcellular platelet factor VIII antigen and von Willebrand factor. J Exp Med 191:1101–1113, 1975.
55. Nachman R, Levine R, Jaffe EA: Synthesis of factor VIII antigen by cultured guinea pig megakaryocytes. J Clin Invest 60:914–921, 1977.
56. Pike GJ, Turner RL, Manohitharajah SM, Deverall PB: Fibrinolysis in cyanotic and acyanotic children before and after open intracardiac operations with Bentley Temptrol oxygenator. J Thorac Cardiovasc Surg 69:922–925, 1975.
57. Quick AJ, Hussey CV: Hemophilic condition in the female (abstract). J Lab Clin Med 42:929–930, 1953.
58. Rand JH, Sussman II, Gordon RE, et al.: Localization of factor VIII-related antigen in human vascular subendothelium. Blood 55:752–756, 1980.
59. Resnekov L, Chediak J, Hirsh J, Lewis D: Antithrombotic agents in coronary artery disease. Chest 89:54S–67S, 1986.
60. Richardson DW, Robinson AG: Desmopressin. Ann Intern Med 103:228–239, 1985.
61. Ruggeri ZM, Mannucci PM, Lombardi R, et al.: Multimeric composition of factor VIII/von Willebrand factor following administration of DDAVP: Implications for pathophysiology and therapy of von Willebrand's disease subtypes. Blood 59:1272–1278, 1982.

62. Ruggeri ZM, Zimmerman TS: The complex multimeric composition of factor VIII/von Willebrand factor. Blood 57:1140–1143, 1981.
63. Sakariassen KS, Cattaneo M, v.d. Berg A, et al.: DDAVP enhances platelet adherence and platelet aggregate growth on human artery subendothelium. Blood 64:229–236, 1984.
64. Salzman EW, Weinstein MJ, Weintraub RM, et al.: Treatment with desmopressin acetate to reduce blood loss after cardiac surgery. N Engl J Med 314:1402–1406, 1986.
65. Solis RT, Beall AC, Noon GP, Debakey ME: Platelet aggregation: Effects of cardiopulmonary bypass. Chest 67:558–563, 1975.
66. Solis RT, Kennedy PS, Beall AC Jr, et al.: Cardiopulmonary bypass: Microembolization and platelet aggregation. Circulation 52:103–108, 1975.
67. Solis RT, Noon P, Beall AC Jr, DeBakey ME: Particulate microembolization during cardiac operation. Ann Thorac Surg 17:332–344, 1974.
68. Stein PD, Collins JJ, Kantrowitz A: Antithrombotic therapy in mechanical and biological prosthetic heart valves and saphenous vein bypass grafts. Chest 89:46S–53S, 1986.
69. Stuart MJ, Ganley C, Reed M, et al.: DDAVP inhibits prostacyclin formation: A potential mechanism for bleeding time correction in hemostatic disorders (abstract). Thromb Haemost 54:151, 1985.
70. Thomas ME, Ormani AH, Scrutton MC: Some properties of the human platelet vasopressin receptor. Thromb Res 32:557–566, 1983.
71. Torosian M, Michelson, EL, Morganroth J, MacVaugh H III: Aspirin and coumadin-related bleeding after coronary artery bypass graft surgery. Ann Intern Med 89:325–328, 1978.
72. Tuddenham EG, Lazarchick J, Hoyer L: Synthesis and release of factor VIII by cultured human endothelial cells. Br J Haematol 47:617–626, 1981.
73. Turitto VT, Weiss HJ, Baumgartner HR: Altered thrombus formation distinct from defective platelet adhesion in von Willebrand's disease (abstract). 62:III–106, 1980.
74. Vincente V, Alberca I, Mannucci PM: High levels of circulating von Willebrand factor inhibit the release of this protein but not of plasminogen activator after DDAVP. Thromb Res 38:101–105, 1985.
75. von Kaulla KN, Swan H: Clotting deviations in man during cardiac bypass: Fibrinolysis and circulating anticoagulants. J Thorac Surg 36:519–526, 1958.
76. Wachtfogel YT, Musial J, Jenkin B, et al.: Loss of platelet α_2-adrenergic receptors during simulated extracorporeal circulation: Prevention with prostaglandin E_1. J Lab Clin Med 105:601–607, 1985.
77. Ware JA, Reaves WH, Horak JK, Solis RT: Defective platelet aggregation in patients undergoing surgical repair of cyanotic congenital heart disease. Ann Thorac Surg 36:289–294, 1983.
78. Watson AJS, Keogh JAB: Effect of 1-deamino-8-D-arginine vasopressin on the prolonged bleeding time in chronic renal failure. Nephron 32:49–52, 1982.
79. Wedemeyer AL, Edson JR, Krivit W: Coagulation in cyanotic congenital heart disease. Am J Dis Child 124:656–660, 1972.
80. Wedemeyer AL, Lewis JH: Improvement in hemostasis following phlebotomy in cyanotic patients with heart disease. J Pediatr 83:46–50, 1973.
81. Weinstein MJ, Salzman EW, Ware JA: Von Willebrand factor multimers during cardiopulmonary bypass: Effect of DDAVP and relation to blood loss (abstract). Blood 68:1251, 1986.
82. Zimmerman TS, Ratnoff OD, Powell AE: Immunologic differentiation of classic hemophilia (factor VIII deficiency) and von Willebrand's disease with observations on combined deficiencies of antihemophilic factor and proaccelerin (factor V) and on an acquired circulating anticoagulant against antihemophilic factor. J Clin Invest 50:244–254, 1971.

CHAPTER 10

THE ACTIVATED COAGULATION TIME (ACT)

CHARLES J. KOPRIVA

The activated coagulation time (ACT) is the hemostatic test most commonly used during cardiac surgery today. Although the coagulation cascade in man is complex, the routine use of the ACT during cardiac surgery is helpful for evaluating the adequacy of anticoagulation during cardiopulmonary bypass (CPB) and for evaluating protamine reversal of heparin. The widespread use of the automated form of this test stems from its ease of performance, low cost, ready availability, and usefulness in evaluating heparin anticoagulation. As with any single coagulation test, the ACT has limitations. However, if used appropriately and interpreted correctly, the ACT can be of tremendous benefit during cardiac surgery.

HISTORY

The ACT was introduced into clinical medicine in 1966 by Hattersley.[1] The technique is a refinement of the Lee-White whole blood coagulation time (WBCT), in which the period of contact activation is markedly decreased by addition of diatomaceous earth to the blood sample. Although Hattersley's motivation for decreasing the period of "contact activation" was to increase the sensitivity of the test as an index of bleeding disorders, it is fortunate that the modifications also made the determination suitable for use in cardiac surgery. Interestingly, the ACT is no longer considered sufficiently sensitive to evaluate or even to screen for bleeding disorders, and today it is used almost exclusively to monitor heparin therapy during cardiac surgery. Ten years after the original description, the manual ACT was introduced into cardiac surgery following a series of articles by Bull.[2-4] Prior to that time, heparin was administered in fixed-dose protocols, which did not allow for individual sensitivity to heparin or for its metabolism. Likewise, protamine reversal of heparinization was usually done empirically, using doses of protamine equal to one to three times the *total* heparin dose. Bull's demonstration of wide variations in heparin sensitivity, together with his method for quantitative heparin administration and protamine reversal, has since gained wide-spread acceptance. Undoubtedly, the quick acceptance of the automated ACT in cardiac surgery was facilitated by ease of performance, by minimal capital expenditure, and, especially, by the fact that the test can be done in the operating room, providing rapid, easily interpretable results.

METHODOLOGY

Performance of an ACT can be done by several different methods. Probably the most common involves the addition of diatomaceous earth to a whole blood sample. Diatomaceous earth is a very fine powder that provides a large surface area, thus accelerating conversion of Factor XII to Factor XIIa. After addition of the diatomaceous earth to the blood sample, the elapsed time until clotting is noted. The exact end point depends upon whether a manual or automated method is being used.

Manual Method

Two cubic centimeters of blood are added to a prewarmed tube containing diatomaceous earth. The tube is shaken vigorously, the timer is started, and the tube is observed over a light box during gentle agitation until the first sign of coagulation occurs. This end point is noted by the decreased ability of the blood to move when the tube is inverted.

Automated Method

The Hemochron 400

Automated methods for the ACT differ from the manual method in several ways. Clotting is detected, and the elapsed time to clotting is recorded automatically, thereby eliminating operator variability. The Hemochron system (manufactured by International Technidyne Corporation, Edison, NJ) utilizes glass tubes containing cylindrical magnets and 12 mg of Celite activator. The device also contains a small magnet detector. The blood sample is added to the prewarmed Hemochron tube, shaken vigorously, and placed into the "well" of the device. The timer is activated, and the tube is slowly rotated. As long as the blood is liquid, the magnet remains in close proximity to the detector at the base of the well. However, when the first strands of fibrin are formed, the magnet becomes enmeshed in fibrin and is displaced away from the detector, tripping a proximity switch that automatically stops the timer, signifying the end point of coagulation.

Although the well of the Hemochron 400 is heated, we have demonstrated that hypothermic blood samples are not warmed to 37° C after placement in the well, resulting in an artificial prolongation of the ACT, independent of heparin levels.[5] However, the manufacturer has constructed a temperature correction nomogram for blood samples ranging from 20° C to 36° C.[13] The Hemochron 400 can be operated by electricity or battery and is completely portable. These features, combined with minimal space requirements, make the device easy to use in the operating room.

The HemoTec Automated ACT System

The HemoTec ACT (manufactured by HemoTec, Inc., Englewood, CO) is a similar device recently introduced which requires only a 0.2 ml blood sample. Automatic clot detection is provided by following the rate of fall of a plastic flag inserted in the blood sample. The device automatically raises the flag to the top of the tube, lets it fall through the blood, and measures the rate of descent. As long as the blood is liquid, the rate of descent is relatively fast. However, when fibrin strands form, the flag falls at a slower pace. This is taken as the end point for the ACT. Since the HemoTec method requires a very small blood sample, it is possible that hypothermic blood samples may have less effect with this device than with larger blood samples as used in the Hemochron. However, this point remains unproven at this time. In addition, experience with this device is limited.

The Hepcon System IV, also manufactured by HemoTec, is a more expensive system that can provide an ACT as part of a more extensive heparin management profile.

THE ACT IN CARDIAC SURGERY

The establishment, maintenance, and reversal of heparin anticoagulation are all extremely important. Failure of heparinization can result from heparin resistance associated with numerous clinical situations or diseases.[6] These are discussed in Chapter 2. Inadequate heparinization can also result from medication errors (i.e., mislabelled drug), variable heparin potency, improper dose, and injection of heparin into a disconnected intravenous line or into a catheter if the portal does not lie within a vein. The routine use of the ACT before the patient is placed on bypass will detect such errors and prevent serious morbidity or mortality. Likewise, the ACT is useful in maintaining adequate anticoagulation during bypass. The "safe" level for ACT during bypass is usually 400 seconds or more. Bypass done at ACT values below 400 seconds results in the appearance of abnormal levels of fibrin monomer and the deposition of fibrin, platelet debris, and cells on the oxygenator.[7] This could lead to disseminated intravascular coagulation (DIC). Proper use of the ACT avoids this problem, as demonstrated by Bull's report of over 3,000 cases without a single incident of DIC.[8]

Although the ACT has been widely accepted, there are theoretical limitations to its use. Culliford et al. have shown that ACT values do not correlate well with heparin levels during *hypothermic* bypass.[9] However, heparin levels are not an end; they are simply a partial means to an end. The desired goal is adequate anticoagulation, which is detected only by the ACT, not by heparin levels. Indeed, heparin levels can be grossly misleading in patients with heparin resistance. In fact, the ACT is a rather precise test of anticoagulation, with a co-efficient of variation of 4.5 to 7 per cent.[10]

Another possible limitation to the use of ACT during hypothermic bypass is the fact that hypothermia exerts a marked additive prolongation of ACT in heparinized patients.[5] The contribution of this additive effect could rapidly disappear during "rewarming," thus leaving the ACT at suboptimal levels. This is not a major problem, however, since the clinician using the Hemochron can use temperature correction factors to predict whether the ACT will fall to unsafe levels during a rapid rewarming[13] (Fig. 10–1). It is necessary to exercise caution in using temperature correction factors when rewarming is done slowly, since heparin metabolism during rewarming may not allow accurate prediction of the normothermic ACT. Frequent serial ACT determinations during the rewarming period are recommended. If the ACT decreases markedly as the blood reaches 30 to 32° C, additional heparin should be administered to ensure adequate anticoagulation during the final minutes of bypass.

PROTAMINE NEUTRALIZATION

In 1975, Bull advocated the quantitative neutralization of heparin by protamine.[3] Using a heparin dose-response curve, it is relatively easy to determine the amount of "circulating" heparin at the end of bypass. According to Bull, administration of protamine (1.3 mg/100 units of

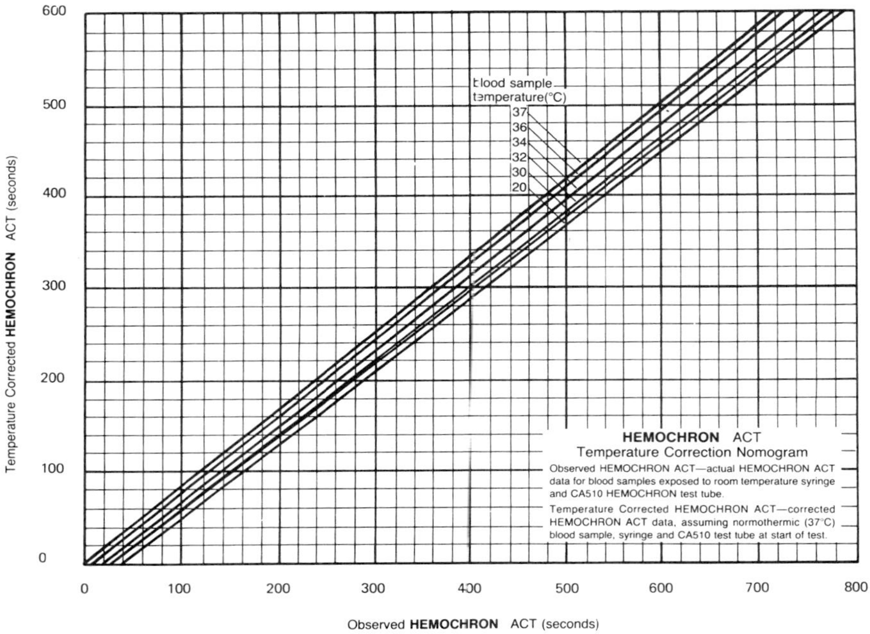

Figure 10–1. Temperature correction nomogram.

circulating heparin/ml) will result in return of the ACT to normal in the vast majority of patients. Mattox also advocated a similar approach for heparin neutralization.[11] However, since blood hypothermia prolongs ACT, independent of heparin levels, it is important that the patient be rewarmed to nearly 37° C before the sample is drawn for calculation of protamine dose. Alternatively, the sample could be drawn at a lower blood temperature, and the temperature correction factors for ACT could be employed. Return of the ACT to preheparinization levels is a very good indication that heparin has been completely neutralized. In a small percentage of cases, the ACT may fail to return to baseline. If so, it is reasonable to slowly administer an additional small dose of protamine (i.e., 50 to 75 mg) to determine if the ACT normalizes. If it does not, the coagulation cascade should be evaluated.[8, 12] Abnormally low procoagulant levels can cause persistent elevation of the ACT despite an adequate protamine dose. Specifically, hypofibrinogenemia may be the cause. Post-pump fibrinogen may be low owing to pump dilution, inadequate heparinization during bypass, or a consumptive coagulopathy following bypass. Patients who were treated with streptokinase and then referred for emergent cardiac surgery may also have post-bypass hypofibrinogenemia (Table 10–1).

Another limitation to the use of the ACT as a hemostatic test following bypass is seen in the patient who continues to bleed despite a normal ACT. Lack of surgical hemostasis is an obvious possibility. If this is not apparent, procoagulant or platelet deficiency may be the cause. The ACT is simply not a sensitive index of qualitative or quantitative platelet abnormalities or of procoagulant deficiency (Table 10–1).[1] This lack of sensitivity explains why the ACT is not used more widely as a screening test.

DETECTION OF HEPARIN REBOUND

Occasionally, cardiac surgical patients will bleed in the Intensive Care Unit secondary to reheparinization. The most sensitive tests for detection of small amounts of heparin are the tri-F titer, protamine titration, and the thrombin/reptilase time combination. Although these tests are sensitive, they take longer to obtain and cost more than an ACT. An alternative first approach is to check the ACT. Postoperative bleeding secondary to reheparinization may be accompanied by a modest ACT elevation. If this is seen, administration of more protamine may be the most practical approach. Return of the ACT to normal and cessation of bleeding confirm the diagnosis.

SUMMARY

The ACT done by automated methods is a simple, inexpensive test that is highly useful in monitoring the adequacy of heparinization during cardiac surgery. Likewise, it is an effective screening test for the adequacy of protamine's neutralization of heparin. It remains the mainstay for routine monitoring of heparin administration and neutralization during cardiac surgery.

TABLE 10–1. PROBLEMS WITH POST-BYPASS USE OF ACT

1. ACT fails to normalize after calculated protamine dose.
   - A. Hypofibrinogenemia
   - B. Other procoagulant deficiency
2. ACT normalizes, but patient continues to bleed.
   - A. Rule out inadequate surgical hemostasis
   - B. Platelet or Factor VII deficiency

References

1. Hattersley PG: Activated coagulation time of whole blood. JAMA 196:150–154, 1966.
2. Bull BS, Huse WM, Brauer FS, Korpman RA: Heparin therapy during extracorporeal circulations. I. Problems inherent in existing protocols. J Thorac Cardiovasc Surg 69:674–684, 1975.
3. Bull BS, Hughes WM, Brauer FS, et al.: Heparin therapy during extracorporeal circulation. II. The use of a dose-response curve to individualize heparin and protamine dosage. J Thorac Cardiovasc Surg 69:685–689, 1975.
4. Bull MH, Hughes WM, Bull BS: Evaluation of tests to monitor heparin therapy during extracorporeal circulation. Anesthesiology 43:346–353, 1975.
5. Kopriva CJ, Sreenivasan N, Stefansson S et al.: Hypothermia can cause errors in activated coagulation time. Anesthesiology 53:S–85, 1980.
6. Anderson EF: Heparin resistance prior to cardiopulmonary bypass. Anesthesiology 64:504–507, 1986.
7. Young JA, Kisker CT, Doty DB: Adequate anticoagulation during cardiopulmonary bypass determined by activated clotting time and the appearance of fibrin monomer. Ann Thorac Surg 26:231–240, 1978.
8. Bull BS: Heparin anticoagulation (letter). Ann Thorac Surg 30:204, 1980.
9. Culliford A, Gitel SG, Starr N, et al.: Lack of correlation between activated clotting time and plasma heparin during cardiopulmonary bypass. Ann Surg 193:105–111, 1981.
10. Doty DB, Knott HW, Hoyt JL, et al.: Heparin dose for accurate anticoagulation in cardiac surgery. J Cardiovasc Surg 70:579–604, 1979.
11. Mattox KL, Guinn GA, Rubio PA, Beall AC: Use of the activated coagulation time in intraoperative heparin reversal for cardiopulmonary operations. Ann Thorac Surg 19:634, 1975.
12. Glass D: The experts opine. Surv Anesth 30:375, 1986.
13. Product information—package insert: Hemochron ACT Tubes Supplied by International Technidyne Corp., 23 Nevsky St., Edison, NJ.

CHAPTER 11

THROMBOELASTOGRAPHY: A Coagulation-Monitoring Technique Applied to Cardiopulmonary Bypass

BRUCE D. SPIESS and ANTHONY D. IVANKOVICH

Thromboelastography (TEG), a qualitative measure of viscoelastic clot strength, was described in 1948 by Hartert.[1] Since then the technique has enjoyed periods of popularity, but has never achieved widespread use in the United States.[2] Recently, TEG has been employed for bedside coagulation monitoring during liver transplantation.[3] Experience gained during this procedure suggests other applications for TEG technology. This chapter will discuss TEG's technical aspects, interpretation of data, correlations with other more routine coagulation data, and use of TEG in perioperative situations, with special reference to cardiopulmonary bypass (CPB) procedures.

TEG PRINCIPLES AND METHODOLOGY

TEG measurements are made using whole or recalcified citrated blood. When using whole blood, the lag time from the drawing of the sample to placement in the TEG machine should be less than 3 minutes to ensure accurate results. A 0.35 ml sample is pipetted into a continuously rotating metal crucible maintained at 37° C. The inside of the crucible is of mirror polished stainless steel; this minimizes clot activation and does not affect either speed of clot formation or breakdown of the blood.[4] A polished metal piston suspended in the blood sample results in a 1 mm annular gap between the piston and the inner wall of the crucible. As clot formation proceeds, fibrin strands form between the wall of the crucible and the suspended piston. As the clot matures, the rotational motion of the crucible is progressively transferred to the piston. An electronic amplification system translates the piston motion into a characteristic TEG tracing (Figs. 11–1 and 11–2). There are two commercially available TEG machines: Biclot Elvi 816 (Logas Scientific, Henderson, NV) and Thrombelastograph Coagulation Analyzer (Haemoscope Corporation, Morton Grove, IL). Both machines are equipped with two channels so that two samples may be run simultaneously. This allows for either temporal sampling or other diagnostic in vitro testing. These options will be discussed later in this chapter.

The characteristic TEG tracing represents the shear elasticity over time of a blood clot as it develops and eventually lyses. A number of parameters can be measured from the TEG tracing (Fig. 11–3). In the operating room, the R, K, α°, MA, and A_{60} measurements are used. The R value (reaction time) is measured from the time of sample placement in the crucible until the TEG tracing amplitude reaches 1 mm; this value represents the time required for initial fibrin formation (normal R = 7.5 to 15 min or 15 to 30 mm).[2, 4-7] Prolongation of the R value may be due to coagulation factor deficiencies, heparin, or severe hypofibrinogenemia.[5-8] A decrease in the R value may be present in hypercoagulability syndromes. The K value (coagulation time) is measured from the R value to the point where the amplitude of the tracing measures 20 mm (normal

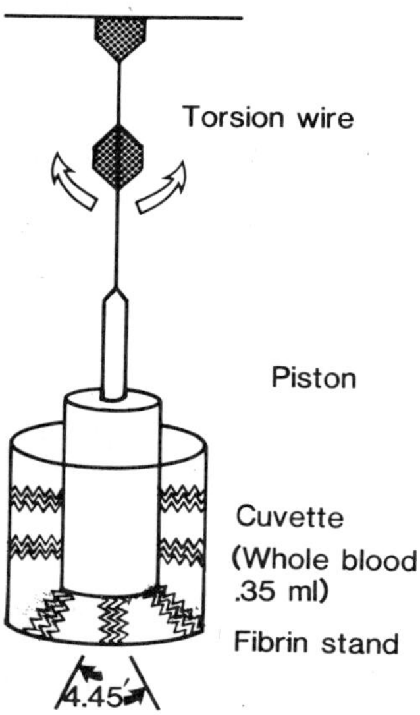

Figure 11–1. The functional components of the TEG consist of a rotating metal cuvette and a suspended piston. As blood in the cuvette coagulates, a connection is completed between the cuvette and the piston, revealing a characteristic tracing over time. (Reprinted with permission from the International Anesthesia Research Society from Effects of progressive blood loss on coagulation as measured by thromboelastography, by Tuman K, Spiess B, McCarthy R, Ivankovich A, Anesthesia Analgesia 66:856–863, 1987.)

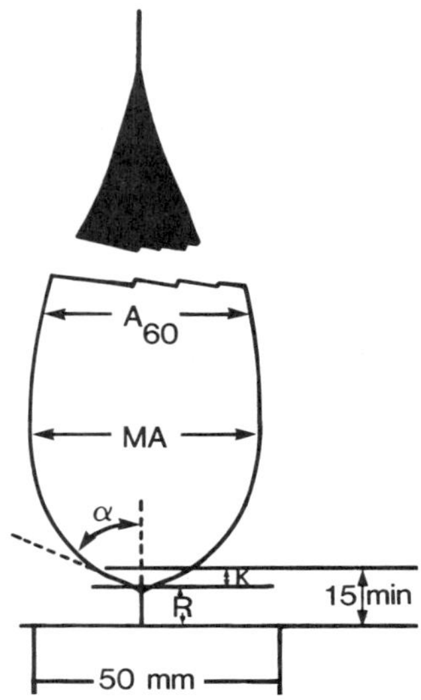

Figure 11–2. A characteristic TEG tracing and standard measurements. Normal values: R = 10 to 15 min, K = 6 to 12 min, $\alpha° = 45°$, MA = 50 to 60 mm, A_{60} = MA − 5 mm; all measurements at 2 mm/min paper speed. (Reprinted with permission from the International Anesthesia Research Society from Effects of progessive blood loss on coagulation as measured by thromboelastography, by Tuman K, Spiess B, McCarthy R, Ivankovich A, Anesthesia Analgesia 66:856–863, 1987.)

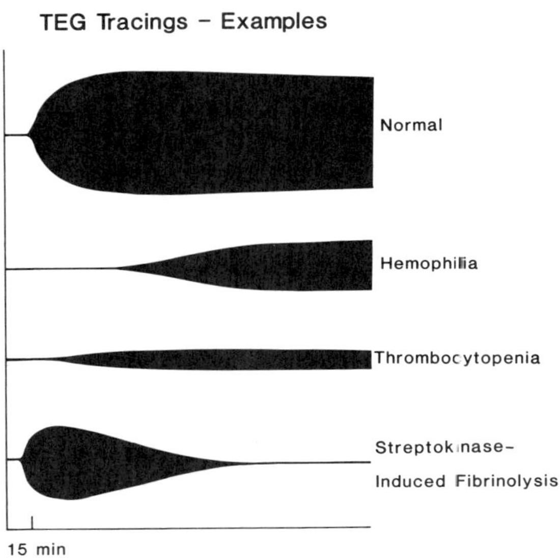

Figure 11–3. Representative abnormal TEG tracings.

K = 3 to 6 min or 6 to 12 mm).[5, 6] The α° is the angle formed by the upslope of the TEG tracing from the R value (normal α° = 45 to 50°).[5, 6] Both the K and the α° angle represent the speed of clot formation, fibrin cross-linking, and platelet-fibrin interaction. Decreased values may occur with hypofibrinogenemia or thrombocytopenia.[5-8] The maximum amplitude (MA) value represents maximum clot strength (normal MA = 50 to 60 mm). Depression of this parameter occurs for the same reasons as depression of the K and α° angle values.[5-8] The A_{60} is the amplitude of the tracing measured 60 minutes after the MA and is a measure of clot retraction or lysis (normal A_{60} = MA − 5 mm).[5, 6] The MA may be very small in cases of disseminated intravascular coagulation (DIC), primary fibrinolysis, and uremia. When activation of clotting is stimulated with cellite, comparisons between the TEG of native blood and the cellite-activated TEG may give an assessment of coagulation reserve.[9, 10]

The data are qualitative, but some specific coagulopathies produce characteristic abnormalities in the tracing (Fig. 11–4). Using a schematic key, abnormal data can be further differentiated to identify etiologies for coagulopathies (Table 11–1). The abnormalities revealed may be treated and/or further diagnosed with other laboratory tests. As a whole blood clotting test, the TEG examines parameters that are interdependent; therefore, abnormalities are rarely isolated to just one parameter of the TEG.[10-13] The key for identifying coagulopathies reflects these interdependencies.

Many studies have compared TEG coagulation data with simultaneously collected routine laboratory test data.[8, 14, 15] Zuckerman et al. reported significant Pearson's R correlation coefficients between the TEG parameter that reflects clot strength (MA) and the fibrinogen level.[14] In a group of patients studied before cardiopulmonary bypass (CPB), there were significant Pearson's R correlations between the R and K values of the TEG and the activated clotting time (ACT) and partial thromboplastin time (PTT) (Table 11–2).[15] Using a different statistical analysis (canonical correlation) with the heaviest weighting placed upon factors related to clot stiffness and overall clot formation, the dominant variables were fibrinogen levels, platelet number, hematocrit, MA, A_{60}, and α° angle.[14] In the CPB population, canonical loading analysis revealed no correlation between TEG values and routine coagulation tests.[15] This discrepancy between bypass and non-bypass patients may be due to medications that affect platelet function given preoperatively to the bypass patients. The populations reported by Zuckerman et al. consisted of healthy, normal volunteers and a group of cancer patients thought to be in a state of hypercoagulability. Tests for clot strength showed the strongest correlations between TEG data and routine test data in the latter group.[14]

TEG has been criticized because of the lack of more highly significant Pearson's R correlations between routine coagulation tests and TEG data

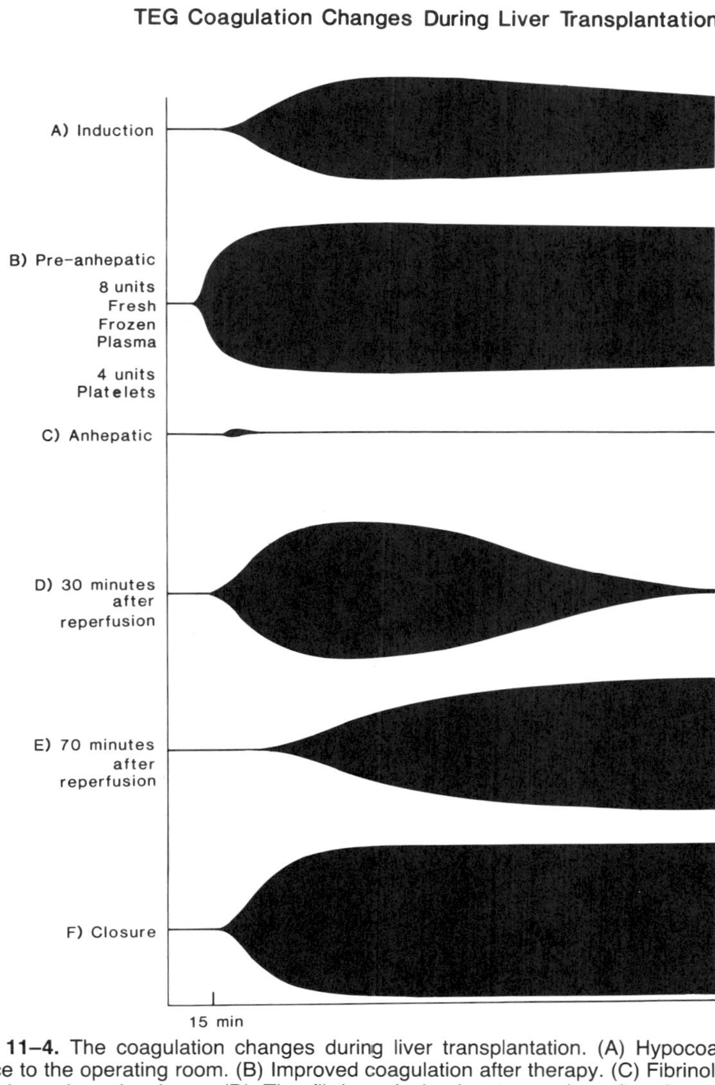

Figure 11–4. The coagulation changes during liver transplantation. (A) Hypocoagulable on entrance to the operating room. (B) Improved coagulation after therapy. (C) Fibrinolysis occurs during the anhepatic phase. (D) The fibrino ysis begins to resolve after the new graft is revascularized. (E and F) Coagulation functior normalizes by closure.

TABLE 11–1. ALGORITHM FOR TEG INTERPRETATION

Data		Interpretation
Normal R + K (20–30 mm)		
MA < 50 MA = A_{60}	(−) (α +)	Thrombocytopenia
MA < 50 R and K	(−) (+)	Hypofibrinogenemia
MA < 50 MA >> A_{60} or A_{60} = 0	(−) (α − −)	Hyperfibrinolysis
Prolonged R + K (Hypocoagulability)		
MA and A_{60} R: + + +, k: +	(n)	Factor V, VII, or X deficient, hepatic failure, or dicumarol treatment
MA = A_{60} R: + + +, k: + + +		Anticoagulant therapy
30 > MA > 20 MA = A_{60}		Thrombocytopenia
MA − A_{60} = 0		Abnormal coagulation with secondary lysis
MA < 20		Heparin treatment or platelet deficiency
MA = 0		Afibrinogenemia or excess heparin
Decreased R + K (Hypercoagulability)		
R: − − K: − A_{60} MA: A_{60}: normal		Plasma-related hypercoagulability
R: − − K: − − − MA: + + +		Platelet-related hypercoagulability
r: − K: − MA: normal, −		Plasma and platelet-related hypercoagulability

in hypocoagulable patients. However, the TEG does not measure the same processes as routine laboratory tests; it examines whole blood coagulation. Thus, the interaction of the protein coagulation cascade, fibrinogen, and the platelet surface are assessed as a total unit. Routine laboratory tests, performed on a centrifuged plasma protein fraction, examine only isolated portions of the coagulation cascade, not the interactions of all the component parts.[16] Although the routine laboratory tests do examine certain links in the coagulation chain, they do not look at interactions among the various factors. It may be unreasonable to expect strict correlations between TEG data and other isolated laboratory tests when the same parameters are not being tested.

TABLE 11–2. PRE-BYPASS CORRELATIONS (PEARSON'S R) COAGULATION TEST FOR TEG PARAMETERS AND OTHER COAGULATION TESTS

TEG PARAMETERS	ACT	PT	PTT	Fib	FS	Plts
R	0.5399*	0.2060	0.6110*	0.0770	0.1594	0.0661
K	0.4862	0.0633	0.0574	0.0378	0.1274	0.0649
Alpha	0.4216	0.0403	0.0502	0.0913	0.2915	0.0093
MA	0.3224	0.1244	0.2211	0.0205	0.0161	0.2468
MA′	0.0759	0.1442	0.0018	0.1541	0.0666	0.2557

*Statistical significance = 0.01

From Spiess B, Tuman K, McCarthy R, et al.: Thromboelastography (TEG) as an indication of post cardiopulmonary bypass coagulopathies. J Clin Monitor 3:25–30, 1987.

PERIOPERATIVE TEG USES

The number of complex and prolonged operations performed in the United States is increasing along with the mean age of the population. Intraoperative coagulation monitoring has historically focused on obtaining multiple different blood tests for routine coagulation monitoring. Samples must often be sent to a remote laboratory for analysis; multiple tests must be conducted to diagnose a coagulation defect. If a crucial laboratory test is not ordered, the defect may be missed or misdiagnosed. There is a need for rapid and complete intraoperative coagulation assessment. The TEG can provide reliable qualitative coagulation data at the bedside or in the operating room in less than 30 minutes. Coagulation replacement therapy can be based on TEG data.[3, 8] In one paper, the authors reported no mortalities associated with massive blood transfusion (> 20 units of blood replaced) in a subsequent 18-month period, after the institution of a coagulation laboratory in the operating room utilizing TEG-guided therapy.[17] Use of TEG-guided therapy reduced bleeding (as well as the need for further blood replacement). This observation, although anecdotal, does point out how a heightened awareness of the need for coagulation monitoring may affect patient outcome. TEG monitoring is easily accessible for the anesthesia/surgical team and heightens vigilance for coagulopathies.

The TEG has gained widespread acceptance for coagulation monitoring during liver transplantation.[3] At the University of Pittsburgh, Kang et al. described more than 66 consecutive liver transplant cases in which the coagulation system was monitored both with routine tests and by TEG. Hepatic failure leads to decreased protein procoagulant synthesis, platelet dysfunction, thrombocytopenia due to splenic sequestration, and possible low-grade DIC fibrinolysis. The orthotopic transplant procedure proceeds through at least three stages: dissection phase, anhepatic phase, and closure phase.[17, 18] Each of these phases has associated metabolic and hemorrhagic derangements that further complicate the pre-existing coagulopathy.[19-21] Transfusion requirements are highly variable, but sudden massive blood loss occurs frequently, requiring replacement of coagulation factors. Without reliable on-site coagulation monitoring guidance, prompt and effective treatment of these complicated clinical situations would be impossible.

Although comparisons of routine laboratory tests with TEG parameters during the stages of liver transplantation show little direct correlation,[3] the TEG tracings often show characteristic changes throughout the stages (Fig. 11–4). Upon the patient's entry into the operating room, the tracing shows a prolonged R value with low K, α°, and MA values, reflecting the overall poor coagulation function of a patient in hepatic failure. After fresh frozen plasma (FFP) and platelet transfusions, the TEG tracing most often shows changes indicative of functional improvement. During the anhepatic phase, TEG tracings consistent with DIC or fibrinolysis may be found. Antiplasmin levels are very low during this phase owing to a lack of hepatic production, and there is no hepatic clearance of activated protein procoagulants. Once the graft is functioning, the DIC clears. By the end of surgery, after administration of cryoprecipitate (CP), platelets, and FFP, the TEG becomes normal. Changes in the patient's coagulation status with component therapy can be easily followed with TEG, particularly if the algorithm discussed earlier is followed for the diagnosis of coagulation deficits. Therapy can then be tailored to the existing clinical situation.

At our institution, we have applied TEG monitoring to a large number of cases in orthopedics, and in general, thoracic, pelvic and neurological surgery. Coagulation changes during the various procedures were followed in 87 adult patients who experienced variable levels of surgical blood loss.[22] All patients received general anesthesia with either isoflurane or halothane in N_2O:O_2. None of the patients had preoperative coagulopathies as diagnosed by PT (prothrombin time), fibrinogen, or platelet counts. At the start of the study no patient was receiving anticoagulants.

Data gathered by TEG reveals a tendency toward a hypocoagulable state after induction of general anesthesia, in comparison with the awake state. The R and K values increase, whereas the α° and MA values decrease (Fig. 11–5). A decrease in circulating "stress" hormones after anesthetic induction may be responsible. Stress has been shown to cause hypercoagulability in both clinical and animal models.[23, 24] A tendency toward hypercoagulability as surgical time progresses may be related to the temporal release of stress hormones and the movement of tissue thromboplastin into the systemic circulation.[25] Hypercoagulability, manifested by decreased R and K values with increased α° and MA values,

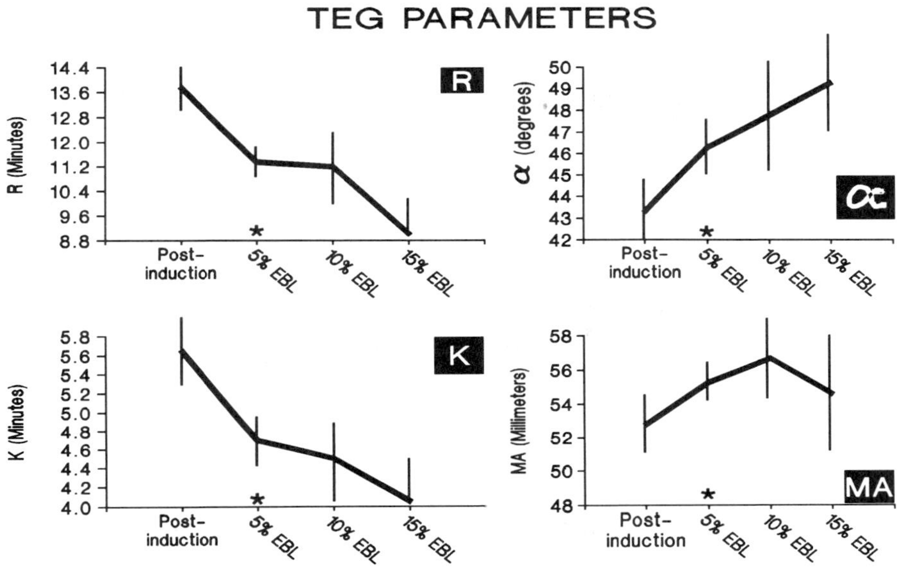

Figure 11–5. The effect anesthesia and mild progressive euvolemic blood have upon TEG parameters. *$p \leq 0.05$ (Reprinted with permission from the International Anesthesia Research Society from Effects of progressive blood loss on coagulation as measured by thromboelastography, by Tuman K, Spiess B, McCarthy R, Ivankovich A, Anesthesia Analgesia 66:856–863, 1987.)

was seen in cases of moderate blood loss and persisted at the conclusion of the operation. The study of coagulation function during progressive blood loss revealed that only patients who had lost 80 per cent of their estimated blood volume showed significant decreases in MA values, along with small decreases in α° values. The changes were attributed to dilutional thrombocytopenia; the MA and α° values normalized after platelet transfusions (Fig. 11–6). Progressive moderate blood loss caused hypercoagulability, not hypocoagulability. In two cases, hypocoagulability was caused by thrombocytopenia, as diagnosed by TEG. Dilutional thrombocytopenia has been noted to be the first change seen in surgical euvolemic hemodilution leading to hypocoagulability.[26, 27] Empirical administration of FFP and platelets after increments of packed red blood cells (RBC's) should be re-evaluated in light of the increasing prevalence of hematologically transmitted diseases, such as acquired immune deficiency syndrome (AIDS) and hepatitis. This euvolemic hemodilution study further demonstrates that TEG can effectively diagnose hypocoagulability states in the operating room during acute blood loss.

TEG can effectively diagnose hypercoagulability preoperatively in

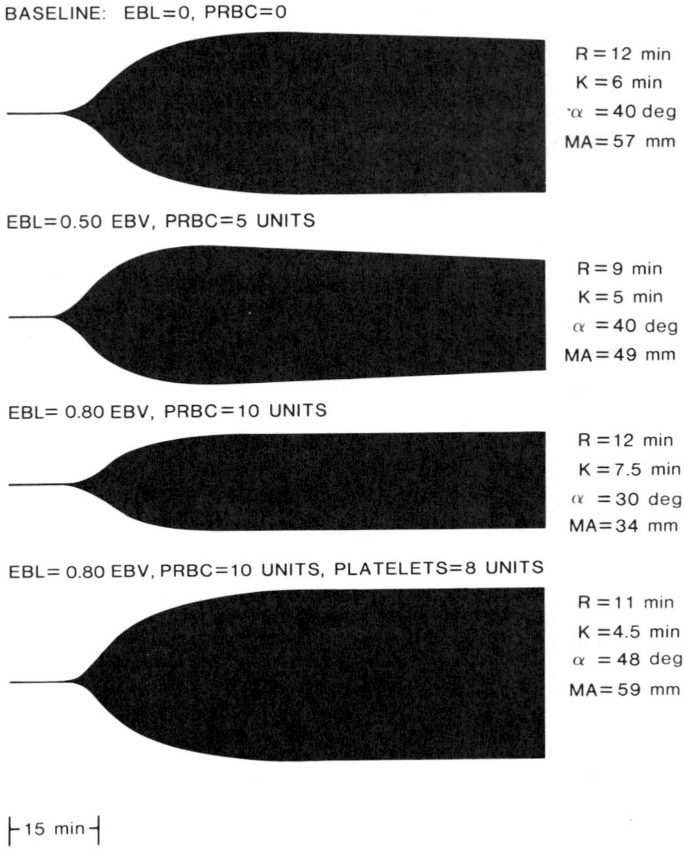

Figure 11–6. TEG tracings sequentially from a patient undergoing progressive major hemorrhage. There is a marked decrease in MA at an 80 per cent estimated blood loss, which probably reflects thrombocytopenia. The TEG tracing normalizes after a platelet transfusion. (Reprinted with permission from the International Anesthesia Research Society from Effects of progressive blood loss on coagulation as measured by thromboelastography, by Tuman K, Spiess B, McCarthy R, Ivankovich A, Anesthesia Analgesia 66:856–863, 1987.)

patients with carcinoma[28, 30–32] and with major vascular disease such as aortic aneurysm.[10, 28–30] Hypercoagulability may occur intraoperatively and postoperatively in a wide range of cases, and may lead to deep venous thrombosis in a significant number of noncardiac operations.[31] Perioperatively, TEG is a very sensitive method for monitoring low-dose heparin therapy, which has been recommended to decrease the incidence of deep venous thrombosis.[33] In these cases, TEG monitoring was reliable and sensitive, and provided more in-depth coagulation data than the activated partial thromboplastin time (aPTT) alone.

Fibrinolysis and DIC may be rapidly diagnosed by TEG.[3, 12, 13] These syndromes occur regularly during liver transplantation and may also occur with massive blood transfusion, CPB, pre-eclampsia, sepsis, amniotic fluid embolism, and in association with fat or air embolism from total joint replacement.[3, 21, 34-36] Routine coagulation testing for DIC and fibrinolysis focuses on the consumption of protein coagulation precursors and the production of fibrin split products.[13, 27] The euglobulin lysis time is a major test for DIC and fibrinolysis. Measurements of the speed of clot lysis by TEG and routine coagulation tests have not been compared for sensitivity and specificity. However, loose correlations are present. If DIC or fibrinolysis is suspected from an abnormal TEG tracing in vitro, a small amount of epsilon-aminocaproic acid (EACA) can be added to the sample before it is placed in the TEG machine.[3, 38] This in vitro test allows one to predict whether systemic EACA therapy will correct the coagulopathy. Administration of EACA may be very dangerous in cases of DIC, but it may be the treatment of choice for isolated fibrinolysis. At our institution, three cases involving fibrinolysis diagnosed by TEG were tested with in vitro EACA before therapy was initiated. Cases included hemorrhage associated with a thoracic tumor resection, aortic aneurysm repair, and renal transplantation. Each patient demonstrated a TEG tracing consistent with fibrinolysis. After in vitro EACA testing, the tracings indicated improvement in coagulation status (Fig. 11–7). Subsequently, each patient was treated with EACA; hemorrhage decreased; and repeat TEG tracings indicated improvements similar to those seen after in vitro testing.

In vitro coagulation testing via TEG and various reagents may be useful in monitoring the effects of streptokinase and urokinase therapy.[13] Dose titration of thrombolytic agents can be individualized with in vitro TEG monitoring, thereby decreasing the hazards of overdosage or ineffective therapy.

The use of TEG for diagnosis of acquired coagulopathies has been discussed previously in this chapter. Perhaps standard in vitro TEG tests could be developed utilizing FFP, platelets, and CP as additives to hypocoagulable blood samples to quantitatively guide transfusion therapy. Such an intraoperative routine would be very useful in reducing the excessive use of some coagulation factor replacement products.

CARDIOPULMONARY BYPASS APPLICATIONS OF TEG

Controlled manipulations of coagulation function are required for successful completion of CPB. Heparin is utilized as the anticoagulant in CPB; its reversal with protamine must be controlled by the anesthesia team. Postoperative hemorrhage is a major cause of morbidity and

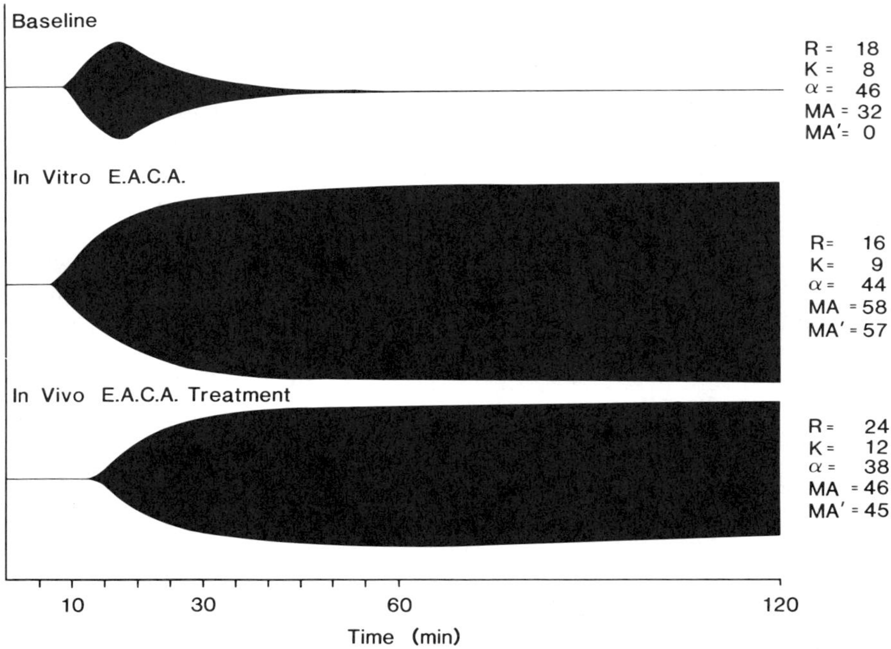

Figure 11–7. Fibrinolysis diagnosed during thoracic tumor resection by TEG. TEG tracings from in vitro EACA testing and treatment of the patient with EACA are displayed.

mortality in post–CPB patients.[39, 40] The effects of hemodilution, along with pump and oxygenator activity, on protein procoagulants, fibrinogen, and platelet number and function have been discussed in other chapters.

Coagulation function and heparin activity during CPB are routinely monitored using activated clotting times or heparin activity assays.[39, 40] The ACT measures the time to initial formation of fibrin and does not correlate with the PTT. The ACT has the advantages of rapid data acquisition, desktop accessibility, and ease of use. The major disadvantage of the ACT is that it assesses coagulation function only up to the time of initial fibrin formation. No information is provided on fibrin-platelet interactions, clot retraction, or clot lysis.[14] Heparin and CPB affect all of these aspects of coagulation; abnormalities will usually result in clinical hemorrhage.

The TEG monitors the interaction of platelets and the coagulation cascade from the onset of clotting through eventual clot lysis. A study of TEG coagulation monitoring during CPB was performed on 38 patients undergoing CPB: 29 had coronary artery bypass grafting (CABG), and 9 had valve replacement operations. Anesthesia and surgical techniques were not altered because of the study. All patients were maintained on their preoperative cardiac medications up to the time of surgery. Blood samples were drawn for ACT, PT, PTT, platelet count, fibrinogen concentration, fibrin split products, and TEG analysis prior to CPB, 45 minutes after the institution of CPB, and 30 minutes after the final administration of protamine. TEG parameters (R, K, α≅, MA, and A_{60} values) were measured from each tracing. Postoperatively, the patients were followed for 24 hours, and chest tube drainage was recorded. Drainage was considered abnormal if it was greater than 1 ml/kg/hr during any 8-hour period. Correlations between TEG parameters and routine coagulation tests were sought for data obtained during the three different collection periods. Abnormal and normal TEG and coagulation test results were analyzed with respect to postoperative bleeding in an attempt to discern if a single value or a specific coagulation profile was an accurate predictor of postoperative hemorrhage.

Thirty minutes following completion of CPB, all ACT's were below baseline levels. One or more standard coagulation tests showed multiple different abnormalities, but no single test consistently showed abnormalities. Of 37 post-bypass patients, TEG tracings in 29 were normal. Eight were abnormal; seven of these had MA values indicative of thrombocytopenia or platelet dysfunction. All of these patients had platelet counts below 100,000/mm^3. One patient had a low A_{60} value indicating fibrinolysis or DIC (Fig. 11–8).

TEG monitoring accurately predicted 80 per cent of postoperative bleeding episodes (Table 11–3). The predictive accuracy of the ACT and the coagulation profile, either together or separately, was 50 per cent or less. The TEG produced false positives (abnormal TEG findings but no abnormal postoperative bleeding) in 20 per cent of cases. There were no false negatives (normal TEG with hemorrhagic diathesis). In one patient, the TEG demonstrated normal clotting function, but the patient had bloody chest drainage. Surgical exploration revealed an arterial bleeding site that had been oversewn. This patient was not included in the data measuring accuracy; in retrospect, the TEG prediction proved accurate. Subsequently, we routinely use TEG monitoring in a large number of CPB cases. TEG is now used whenever a patient develops bleeding in the early postoperative period. The data obtained are instrumental in deciding whether to re-explore for surgical hemorrhage. Guidance of coagulation replacement therapy with TEG in the intensive care unit provides reassurance that therapy is improving an existing coagulopathy.

Correlations between the routine coagulation tests and TEG parameters have been discussed earlier in this chapter (see Table 11–2). Although loose correlations exist in the pre-bypass period between routine coagulation tests and TEG data, no correlations are found in the post-bypass period. Weak correlations in the pre-bypass period may be related to the

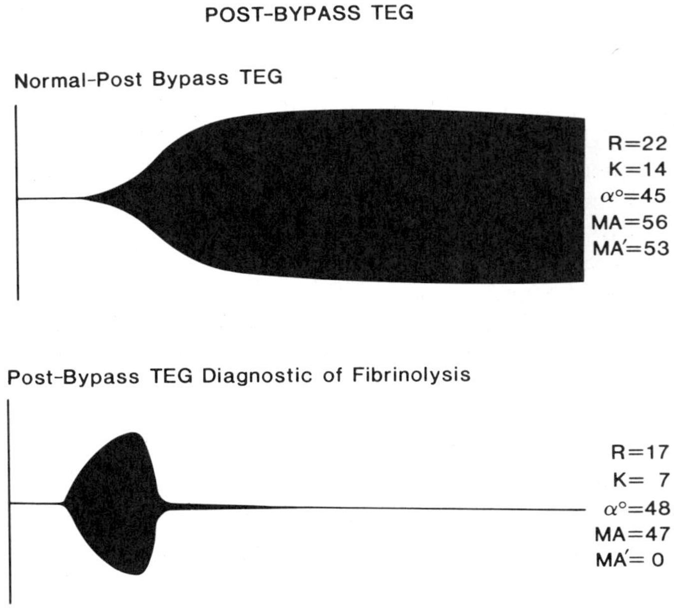

Figure 11–8. Fibrinolysis in a patient after cardiopulmonary bypass. (From Spiess B, Tuman K, McCarthy R, et al.: Thromboelastography (TEG) as an indication of post cardiopulmonary bypass coagulopathies. J Clin Monitor 3:25–30, 1987.)

effect of these cardiac patients' medications on platelets. In the post-bypass period, it is reasonable to expect that correlations should not exist. The TEG measures the interaction of the platelet surface with the coagulation cascade as whole blood clotting proceeds. CPB changes platelet surface activity and platelet myofibrillar contraction; routine plasma fraction coagulation tests do not assess such changes in the interactions of the protein cascade with platelets.

TABLE 11–3. PREDICTIVE ACCURACY FOR POSTOPERATIVE HEMORRHAGE

	TEG	ACT	Coagulation Profile
Percentage correct prediction	80*	40	30
Percentage false positive	20*	50	70
Percentage false negative	0	10	0

*Statistical significance ($p \leq 0.05$)

From Spiess B, Tuman K, McCarthy R, et al.: Thromboelastography (TEG) as an indication of post cardiopulmonary bypass coagulopathies. J Clin Monitor 3:25–30, 1987.

Many CPB patients receive aspirin and dipyridamole as platelet function inhibitors immediately prior to surgery. ACT and heparin assay tests performed intraoperatively will not assess platelet function. When platelet function is affected by aspirin or dipyridamole, or in the case of thrombocytopenia, the TEG will show a decreased MA value. It is very important to evaluate platelet function in CPB patients after bypass, especially in the patient subgroup that has received aspirin and dipyridamole. Intraoperative platelet function testing by routine coagulation tests is impractical. ADP-stimulated function tests are labor- and time-intensive and expensive and are not available 24 hours a day in coagulation laboratories. Template bleeding times are not practical for use in the operating room setting. However, data on both platelet number and function can be obtained by TEG analysis.

At our institution, a protocol is followed whereby patients demonstrating abnormal bleeding and abnormal TEG findings will have TEG-directed therapy; the TEG will have to return to "normal" before surgical re-exploration is considered. Patients who have deteriorating vital signs are exempt and are immediately re-explored. The use of postoperative TEG-guided therapy is being studied now with respect to reoperation rate and utilization of FFP and platelets. Preliminary results mirror those found in the original CPB and TEG study, in terms of TEG's ability to predict post–CPB bleeding and its lack of correlation with routine coagulation tests. Utilization of TEG in the immediate post-bypass period should not be at the exclusion of all other laboratory testing. However, we feel comfortable in guiding therapy by TEG for the following reasons: (1) rapid return of results, (2) high predictive accuracy for hemorrhage, (3) ability to assess the platelet-protein polymer interaction, (4) easy detection of DIC and fibrinolysis, (5) heightened sensitivity to heparin-induced hypocoagulability states, (6) unique ability to detect hypercoagulability states, (7) ease of use, and (8) cost containment due to reusable components. The lack of correlation between routine coagulation tests and the TEG, in conjunction with the predictive accuracy of TEG for postoperative hemorrhage, forms a very strong argument for TEG's routine use throughout CPB.

During CPB, TEG is not useful for assessing the adequacy of heparinization during the bypass run. TEG is far too sensitive to heparin; even low levels will produce a straight-line tracing. Conversely, if any TEG tracing is found during CPB, an antithrombin-III deficiency, heparin antibody presence, or mechanical problem with heparin administration should be suspected. Low-dose heparin therapy can be followed adequately with the TEG, but quantitative assessment of heparinization for bypass cannot be made with this technique.

1-Deamino-8-D-arginine vasopressin (demopressin acetate, or DDAVP)

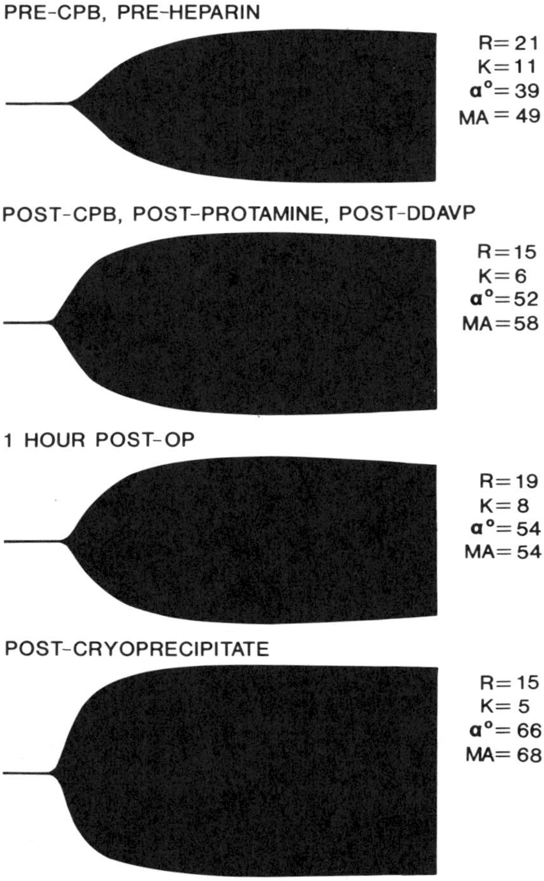

Figure 11–9. TEG tracings from a patient with von Willebrand's disease undergoing CPB, demonstrating the effects of DDAVP and CP treatments. (From Tuman K, Spiess B, McCarthy R, Ivankovich A: Use of thromboelastography in the management of von Willebrand's disease during TEG in cardiopulmonary bypass. J Cardiothoracic Anesth 1:321–324, 1987.)

increases certain fractions of Factor VIII (von Willebrand's factor) and promotes platelet adhesiveness. Desmopressin acetate has been used in uremic patients and in patients with von Willebrand's disease. It may also act as a mild plasminogen activator. Recent reports of desmopressin administration during CPB linked its use with decreased postoperative bleeding.[41] One patient with known von Willebrand's disease was followed during CPB and desmopressin therapy with TEG monitoring.[42] The TEG tracing provided complementary qualitative routine laboratory tests, and demonstrated the effects of desmopressin therapy in the post-bypass period (Fig. 11–9). As future protocols involving desmopressin acetate are designed for use in CPB, TEG monitoring should prove instructive for coagulation monitoring.

TEG monitoring is uniquely suited for monitoring coagulation function in the operating room, and its future appears bright. As anesthesiologists gain exposure to TEG and become familiar with interpretation of the tracings, it will be more extensively applied not only in liver transplantation and CPB, but in all types of surgeries. Empirical or "shotgun" coagulation therapy is unwise. We must be able to justify any administration of blood or blood components. The Centers for Disease Control have reported that FFP, a vector for many viral diseases, is the most inappropriately utilized blood product. TEG monitoring should allow rational application of coagulation therapy, including the use of blood products. Perhaps anesthesiologists could safely proceed with regional anesthetic procedures when the TEG is normal. Hypercoagulability caused by surgical trauma (tissue thromboplastins and stress) or preexisting disease can be uniquely diagnosed by TEG. Deep venous thrombosis, pulmonary embolism, coronary artery and artificial graft thrombosis, as well as hepatic artery thrombosis, are all complications of hypercoagulability. Future therapeutic protocols may identify patient groups at risk for hypercoagulability; monitoring with TEG perioperatively may decrease the incidence of thrombotic and thromboembolic complications. Toward this end, advanced techniques for assessing hypercoagulability and coagulation reserve have been proposed utilizing cellite clot activation in conjunction with TEG monitoring.[9, 32] Comparison of cellite clot activation data and native whole blood TEG data may be a method for assessing coagulation reserve in CPB. The use of in vitro testing, such as that already demonstrated for EACA, may be increased. Linkage with the computer software and hardware being developed will allow for automatic measurement and analysis of TEG data.

Although TEG is not a new monitoring technique, it is one that is now gaining acceptance by anesthesiologists. It has proved invaluable in liver transplantation and is particularly suited for the needs of the operating room, where clot strength, speed of clot formation, and clot breakdown provide critical information for anesthesiologists. Abnormal PT's or aPTT's tell us little about the speed of clot formation, maximum clot strength, or lytic activity; these measurements describe what happens in an isolated plasma fraction stimulated to clot formation in vitro. Specificity for factor analysis is occasionally necessary, but the clinician in the operating room is benefitted more by the guidance of a rapid on-site qualitative test such as the TEG. CPB and multiple other surgical endeavors will be made safer for patients in the future with the progressive extensive application of TEG coagulation monitoring.

References

1. Hartert H: Blutgerinnung studien mit der thrombelastographie, einen neuen untersuchingsverfahren. Klin Wochenschr 26:577–583, 1948.
2. Hartert H, Schaeder JA: The physical and biological constants of thromboelastography. Biorheology 1:31–39, 1962.
3. Kang YG, Martin D, Marquez J, et al.: Intraoperative changes in blood coagulation and thrombelastographic monitoring in liver transplantation. Anesth Analg 64:888–897, 1985.
4. Carr SH, Zuckerman L, Caprini JA, Vagher JP: In vitro testing of surface thrombogenecity using the thromboelastograph. Res Commun Chem Pathol Pharmacol 13:507–519, 1976.
5. Thromboelastograph operator's manual. Logos Scientific, Henderson, Nevada.
6. Thrombelastograph D; operation manual. Hellige GMBH 1979, West Germany, 1979.
7. DeNicola P, Mazzetti GM: Evaluation of thrombelastography. Am J Clin Pathol 25:447–451, 1955.
8. Howland WS, Schweizer O, Gould P: Comparison of intraoperative measurements of coagulation. Anesth Analg 53:657–663, 1974.
9. Caprini JA, Zuckerman L, Cohen E, et al.: The identification of accelerated coagulability. Thromb Res 9:167–180, 1980.
10. Howland WS, Castro EB, Fortner JB, Gould PG: Hypercoagulability: thrombelastographic monitoring during extensive hepatic surgery. Arch Surg 108:605–608, 1974.
11. de Gaetano G, Bottclia D, Vernylen J: Effect of platelets on clot structuration: a thrombelastographic study. Thromb Res 3:425–435, 1973.
12. Astrys T, Egeblad K: Thrombelastographic patterns produced by fibrinolytic agents incorporated in fibrin. Am J Physiol 209:84–94, 1965.
13. Summaria L, Sandesara J, Yang G, et al.: In vitro comparison of fibrinolytic activity of plasminogen activators using a thromboelastographic method: In-vivo evaluation of the B-chain streptokinase complex in the dog model using pre-titered doses. Thromb Haemost November, 1147–1163, 1986.
14. Zuckerman L, Cohen E, Vagher JP, et al.: Comparison of thromboelastography with common coagulation tests. Thromb Haemost 46:752–756, 1981.
15. Spiess B, Tuman K, McCarthy R, et al.: Thromboelastography (TEG) as an indication of post–cardiopulmonary bypass coagulopathies. J Clin Monit 3:25–30, 1987.
16. Miale JB: Laboratory Medicine: Haemotology. St. Louis, CV Mosby, 1977.
17. Starzl JE, Koep LJ, Halgmason LG, et al.: Fifteen years of clinical liver transplantation. Gastroenterology 77:375–388, 1979.
18. Farman JV: Anesthesia in the presence of liver disease and hepatic transplantation. Br J Anaesth 44:946–949, 1972.
19. Borland LM, Marena R, Cook DR: Anesthesia for pediatric orthotopic liver transplantation. Anesth Analg 64:117–124, 1985.
20. Howland WS, Ryan G, Bettigole R, Fortwer J: Coagulation abnormalities associated with liver transplantation. Surgery 68:591–596, 1970.
21. Carmichael FJ, Lindop MJ, Faman MB: Anesthesia for hepatic transplantation. Anesth Analg 64:108–116, 1985.
22. Tuman K, Spiess BD, McCarthy R, Ivankovich AD: Effects of progressive blood loss on coagulation as measured by thrombelastography. Anesth Analg 66:856–863, 1987.
23. Miller RD, Robbins TO, Tong MJ, et al.: Coagulation defects associated with massive blood transfusions. Ann Surg 174:794, 1971.
24. Miller RD: Complications of massive blood transfusions. Anesthesiology 39:82, 1973.
25. Mannucci PM, Gagnatell G, D'alonzo R: Stress and blood coagulation. In Briukhous K (ed): Thrombosis. Schattauer, Stuttgart, 1972, p. 105.
26. Gader AMA, Clarkson AR, Cash JD: The plasminogen activator and coagulation factor VIII response to adrenaline, noradrenaline, isoprenoline and sulbutanol in man. Thromb Res 2:9, 1979.
27. Butler MJ, Britton BJ, Smith M, et al.: Coagulation and fibrinolytic responses during operative surgery. Br J Surg 62:8, 1975.

28. Raina S, Spillert C, Greenstein S, Lazaro E: Effect of surgery on tumor-induced accelerated coagulation in a rat carcinoma. J Surg Res 38:138–142, 1985.
29. Caprini JA, Zuckerman L, Cohen E, et al.: The identification of accelerated coagulability. Thromb Res 9:167–180, 1976.
30. Jennings S, Cass A, Heather B, Greenhalgh R: Coagulation changes during major surgery and relationship to post-operative deep vein thrombosis. J Cardiovasc Surg 22:327–329, 1981.
31. Amundsen MA, Spittel JA, Thompson JH, Owen CA: Hypercoagulability associated with malignant disease and with postoperative state: Evidence for elevated levels of antihemophilic globulin. Ann Intern Med 58:608–616, 1963.
32. Cohen E, Caprini J, Zuckerman L, et al.: Evaluation of three methods used to identify accelerated coagulability. Thromb Res 10:587–604, 1977.
33. Eliot R, Von Kaulla K, Blount SG: Thrombelastographic studies with a twenty-four-hour schedule for subcutaneous heparin. Circulation 24:1206–1214, 1961.
34. Bonnar J, McNicol GP, Douglas AS: Coagulation and fibrinolytic mechanics during and after normal childbirth. Br Med J 2:200–203, 1970.
35. Bachman F, McKenna ER, Cole J, Najafi H: The hemostatic mechanism after open-heart surgery. J Thorac Cardiovasc Surg 70:76–85, 1975.
36. Stibbe J, Kluft C, Brommer EJP, et al.: Enhanced fibrinolytic activity during cardiopulmonary bypass in open-heart surgery in man is caused by extrinsic (tissue type) plasminogen activation. Eur J Clin Invest 14:357–382, 1984.
37. Bell WR, Meck AG: Guidelines for the use of thrombolytic agents. N Engl J Med 301:1266–1270, 1979.
38. Spiess B, Logas W, Hughes T, Ivankovich AD: Perioperative fibrinolysis as diagnosed by thrombelastography: A report of three cases (submitted for publication).
39. Bick RL: Hemostasis defects associated with cardiac surgery, prosthetic devices and other extracorporeal circuits. Semin Thromb Hemost 11:249–280, 1985.
40. Mammen E, Koets M, Washington B, et al.: Hemostasis changes during cardiopulmonary bypass surgery. Semin Thromb Hemost 11:281–292, 1985.
41. Salzman EW, Weinstein MJ, Weintraub RM, et al.: Treatment with desmopressin acetate to reduce blood loss after cardiac surgery: A double-blind randomized trial. N Engl J Med 314:1402–1406, 1986.
42. Tuman K, Spiess B, McCarthy R, Ivankovich AD: Use of thromboelastography in the management of von Willebrand's disease during cardiopulmonary bypass. J Cardio Thoracic Anesth 1:321–324, 1987.

CHAPTER 12

VISCOELASTIC MEASUREMENT OF CLOT FORMATION: The Sonoclot

SALWA A. SHENAQ and ABDUS SALEEM

At present, a reasonable proficiency has been achieved in evaluating the components of hemostasis. Whole blood clotting has not received much attention since the classic test of whole blood clotting time fell into disfavor because of the lack of precision and accuracy.[1] Modifications to improve the precision and acceptability of this measurement led to evaluation of blood components rather than of total clotting. This chapter describes a way of measuring blood clotting as a whole.

The search for a device to measure the coagulation of blood started in 1889, when Hayem suggested changes in viscosity as a test of blood coagulation.[2] In 1894, Wright added temperature control during the determination of clotting time by placing a capillary tube in a water bath at 15° C.[3] In 1913, Lee and White recommended that blood obtained by venipuncture be used for the measurement of coagulability, rather than capillary blood, which they considered to be unreliable.[4] Until 1910 the continuous measurement of coagulation was infeasible. By introducing his coaguloviscosimeter, Koffman was the first to attempt continuous measurement of changes in blood viscosity during coagulation.[5] Many technical improvements have been made to his device since its introduction. In 1923, Kugelmass introduced a second viscosimeter, which formed the basis for the modern thromboelastograph.[6] Von Kaulla, in 1975, described a device (Sonoclot, manufactured by Sienco, Inc., Morrison, CO) that assesses coagulation by changes in impedance.[7] The characteristics of this desirable bedside coagulation screening device are shown in Table 12–1.

TABLE 12–1. CHARACTERISTICS OF A DESIRABLE BEDSIDE COAGULATION SCREENING DEVICE

1. Whole blood or plasma can be used.
2. Device can be adapted to small volumes of specimen (0.05 ml or less).
3. Coagulation process can be observed (transilluminated specimen).
4. Blood or plasma remains practically undisturbed.
5. It writes real-time curves, providing a permanent record.
6. Device produces continuous electric signal.
7. It records long (minutes to hours) and short (seconds) clotting processes.
8. Only disposable elements come in contact with blood or plasma.
9. The device is simple, compact, sturdy, portable, and thermostatically controlled.
10. Easy to start, runs by itself, and requires little servicing.
11. Its sensitivity and characteristics are adjustable to meet specific test requirements.
12. It can be used with most commercial recorders.

(Reproduced with kind permission from PJD Publications Limited, Westbury, NY, 11590, USA, adapted from Von Kaulla KN, Ostendorf P, Von Kaulla E: The impedance machine: A new bedside coagulation recording device. J Med 6:73–87, 1975. Copyright by PJD Publications Ltd.)

METHODOLOGY

Technique

The Sonoclot (Fig. 12–1) uses a plastic vibrating probe immersed to a fixed depth in either whole blood or plasma. The amount of fluid required is 0.4 ml. The frequency of probe vibration is approximately 200 Hz.[8] The blood or plasma exerts a resistance or impedance to the movement of the probe in proportion to the viscosity. The impedance is detected by the driving electronic circuit, which in turn converts this impedance into an output signal. The magnitude of the signal will be directly

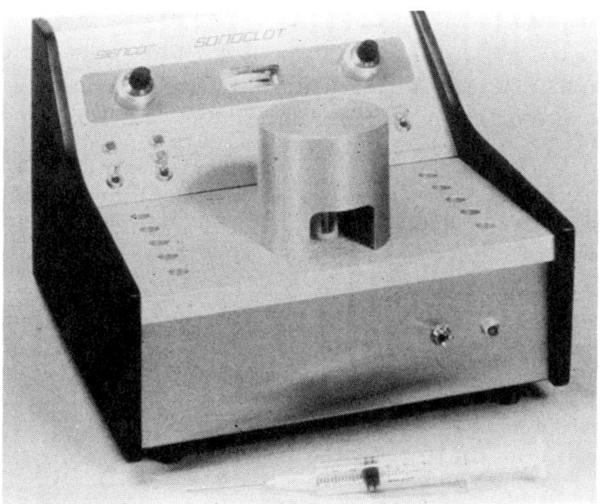

Figure 12–1. The Sonoclot Coagulation Analyzer Model DP-154.

proportional to the fluid's viscoelasticity. This will exert impedance upon the vibrating probe, leading to an increased output signal that will be recorded using a time-based strip chart recorder into which the signal is fed. The recorder will provide a "signature" of the entire clotting, clot retraction, and clot lysis processes.

The blood is collected in 3.8 per cent sodium citrate solution, maintaining a blood-to-citrate ratio of 9:1. Plasma from this sample is recalcified in the cuvette with the addition of 0.2 ml of $CaCl_2$ (0.5 molar). The 0.4 ml specimen of whole blood can be used without further processing. If platelet-rich plasma (PRP) is desired, the specimen is spun at 100 g for 10 minutes, and supernatant PRP is removed for the test. For platelet-poor plasma (PPP), the PRP may be spun at 1000 g for 15 minutes. Supernatant PPP is removed for the test. Table 12–2 lists normal values for PRP and PPP.

Interpretations

Signature (Fig. 12–2). The lag phase (A) represents the recalcification time. The primary wave (B) depicts the rate of conversion of fibrinogen into fibrin. The shoulder (C) separates the secondary wave (D), which represents the increase in viscosity of clot during isometric clot retraction.

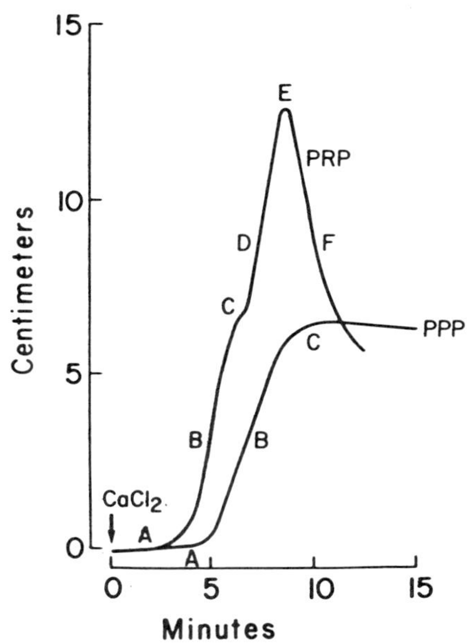

Figure 12–2. Comparison of clot impedance of platelet-rich plasma (PRP) and platelet-poor plasma (PPP). A = Lag period; B = primary wave; C = shoulder; D = secondary wave; E = peak; F = downward wave. (From Saleem A, Blifeld C, Saleh SA, et al.: Viscoelastic measurement of clot formation: A new test of platelet function. Ann Clin Lab Sci 13:115–124, 1983.)

The clot is still in contact with the probe and the sides of the cuvette. As the clot retracts, first from the bottom and then from the sides of the cuvette, the probe and clot become one vibrating structure in a less viscous medium, the serum. This results in a "decrease" of viscosity and a downward deflection (F).

Whole Blood or Platelet-Rich Plasma (Fig. 12–2). Following recalcification, there is a lag period (A) of 3.5 min when the chart tracing is at the baseline. As the clot formation starts, the tracing shows the primary wave (B), followed by a shoulder (C) and the secondary wave (D); at about 6 to 10 min following recalcification, the secondary wave reaches a peak (E), and a downward deflection (F) follows.

Platelet-Poor Plasma (Fig. 12–2). The signature of PPP differs from that of PRP or whole blood in having a lag phase and primary wave only. After the primary wave, the tracing plateau does not show any secondary wave or downward deflection.

Although exact determinants of all phases of the tracings are not very well understood, the basis of the impedance changes can be postulated, and some of the findings can be correlated with the clinical setting. The tracing from the PPP is distinctly different from that of the PRP. The lag period of PPP is longer, and the slope of the primary wave is less steep than that of PRP. In addition, the tracing of PPP shows a plateau after the primary wave but no secondary wave or downward deflection. This apparently indicates that all fibrinogen has been converted to fibrin by the end of the primary wave in PPP signatures. No further fibrin formation, isometric contraction, or retraction of clot occurs in PPP. Conversely, signatures of PRP demonstrate distinct lag phase, primary and secondary wave, and downward deflection. The last two phases represent the isometric contraction and retraction of clot from the sides or bottom of the cuvette. Table 12–2 compares the normal values obtained from PPP and PRP signatures.

TABLE 12–2. SONOCLOT VALUES OF PLATELET-POOR PLASMA AND PLATELET-RICH PLASMA

	Lag Period (sec)	Primary Wave Slope (cm/min)	Secondary Wave Slope (cm/min)	Shoulder-Peak Interval (sec)
Platelet-poor plasma	550 ± 105	1.2 ± 0.3	—	—
Platelet-rich plasma	330 ± 45*	2.3 ± 0.5*	3.5 ± 0.6	180 ± 30

Note: All values are expressed as mean ± SD.

*Compared with platelet-poor plasma, $p < 0.01$.

(From Saleem A, Blifeld C, Saleh SA, et al.: Viscoelastic measurement of clot formation: A new test of platelet function. Ann Clin Lab Sci 13:115–124, 1983.)

We have demonstrated that signatures of PRP are dependent on the number of platelets (Fig. 12–3). It is apparent that (1) as platelet count of PRP increases, the lag phase decreases, (2) slopes of primary and secondary waves increase, (3) shoulder-peak interval decreases, and (4) downward deflection becomes prominent. It may be noted that the secondary wave first appears within a platelet count of 30,000/mm^3 and the downward deflection appears at about 60,000/mm^3.

The signatures of PRP also depend on the quality of functioning platelets. For example, 8-day-old PRP with a platelet count of 250,000/cu mm produces a signature similar to that of PPP. Also, sonication of PRP, which destroys the integrity of platelets, produces a signature resembling that of PPP.

CLINICAL APPLICATIONS

Following Cardiopulmonary Bypass (CPB)

Bleeding in patients after CPB surgery remains a serious complication. The cause of excessive bleeding may be surgical, hemostatic failure, or a combination of both. Several recent studies have emphasized the importance of platelet function defects following CPB surgery.[9] Although recent technology in clotting provides valuable information on coagulation factors, the platelet dysfunction tests are insensitive. The platelet count

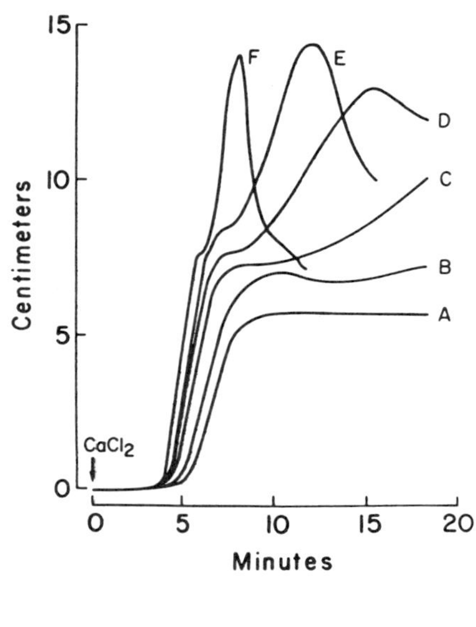

Figure 12–3. Effect of increasing concentration of platelets on Sonoclot tracings. A = Platelet-poor plasma; B = 15 K/μl; C = 30 K/μl; D = 60 K/μl; E = 88 K/μl; F = 250 K/μl. (From Saleem A, Blifeld C, Saleh SA, et al.: Viscoelastic measurement of clot formation: A new test of platelet function. Ann Clin Lab Sci 13:115–124, 1983.)

TABLE 12–3. POSTOPERATIVE CLINICAL AND LABORATORY DATA ON 69 PATIENTS AFTER CORONARY ARTERY BYPASS SURGERY

	Pump Time (min)	Maximum Post-op Blood Loss (ml/hr)	Platelet Count (K/μl)	Template Bleeding Time (min)
Normal Range	N/A	N/A	275 ± 60	5.0 ± 1.5
Controls				
Group A (n = 20)	68 ± 10	60 ± 15	200 ± 38†	5.2 ± 1.5
Group B (n = 24)	75 ± 15	405 ± 130*	223 ± 48†	4.6 ± 2.0
Group C (n = 25)	76 ± 18	262 ± 60*	116 ± 25*†	8.0 ± 4.2*

Note: All values are expressed as mean ± 1 SD.
*$p < 0.01$ compared with controls.
†$p < 0.01$ compared with normal.

provides a numerical, but not a qualitative, index. Template bleeding time is subject to wide variations. Platelet aggregation tests are time-consuming.[8]

We used this device along with routine coagulation tests to determine if bleeding was the result of hemostatic failure. Forty-nine patients who had excessive bleeding after CPB surgery and 20 controls formed the study group. The 49 CPB patients were divided into two groups: group B (24 patients), in which patients showed no signature abnormalities, and group C (25 patients), in which patients had abnormal signatures (Table 12–3).

Comparison of patients in group B with those in control group A showed significantly greater bleeding per hour in the former group. The platelet count, the lag, the primary and secondary waves, and the shoulder-peak interval did not show statistical significance. The prothrombin time (PT) and partial thromboplastin time (PTT) were normal in group B. A diagnosis of adequate medical hemostasis was made, and the patients were surgically explored. In 22 of 24 patients, one or more bleeding vessels were found. These vessels were ligated, resulting in satisfactory hemostasis.

Compared with the control group, patients in group C also showed a significantly higher rate of bleeding per hour, and signatures were abnormal. These patients received 10 units of platelet concentrate. In 18 of 25 patients, the bleeding was controlled within 30 minutes of platelet

	Sonoclot Parameters			
	Lag (sec)	*Primary Wave Slope (cm/min)*	*Secondary Wave Slope (cm/min)*	*Shoulder-peak Time (sec)*
Normal Range	330 ± 45	2.3 ± 0.5	3.5 ± 0.5	180 ± 30
Controls				
Group A (n = 20)	348 ± 60	2.0 ± 0.6	3.0 ± 0.8	200 ± 37
Group B (n = 24)	355 ± 57	2.2 ± 0.7	3.2 ± 0.6	190 ± 45
Group C (n = 25)	450 ± 60*	1.5 ± 0.6*	1.7 ± 0.4*	325 ± 40*

(From Saleem A, Blifeld C, Saleh SA, et al.: Viscoelastic measurement of clot formation: A new test of platelet function. Ann Clin Lab Sci 13:115–124, 1983.)

transfusion. In 3 of 25 patients, the bleeding tapered but was controlled in 2 hours. In the remaining 4 patients, the bleeding continued and surgical exploration did not reveal any localized bleeding. The bleeding ultimately tapered off in 4 to 12 hours after exploration. The signatures returned to normal in all patients in group C after platelet transfusion.

Scanning electron micrographic studies on one of the patients with severe bleeding after CPB showed globular platelets with little pseudopod formation and poor attachment of the platelets to fibrin. (Fig. 12–4 shows normal platelet function; Fig. 12–5 shows abnormal platelet function.) We concluded that signatures provided predictable information regarding platelet function after CPB surgery.[8]

In Hypercoagulable States

In 1979 Peck evaluated viscoelastic measurements for detection of hypercoagulable states in 67 normal subjects and 486 patients.[10] Other laboratory tests performed included PT, thrombin generation test (TGT), activated partial thromboplastin time (aPTT), antithrombin-III (AT-III), and platelet count. Signatures were obtained on PPP after recalcification to eliminate the contribution of platelets to the signature. The lag time, primary slope, and the time to reach the peak were recorded. On the basis of their clinical presentation, the patients were divided into five groups classified on a scale of 0 to 4, where 0 = normal and 4 = clinical evidence of thromboembolism. Peck reported a sensitivity of 57 to 100 per cent detection for TGT and 64 to 67 per cent detection of signature in the high-risk group (groups 3 and 4). A combination of these two tests gave a sensitivity of 79 to 100 per cent detection. The false-positive rate

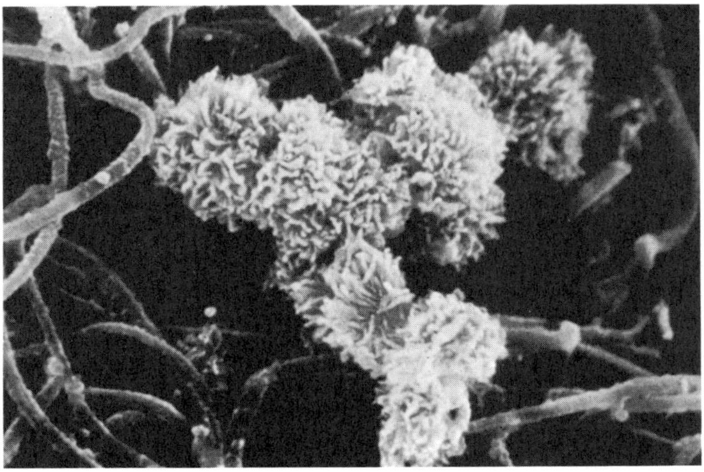

Figure 12–4. Scanning electron micrograph of recalcified normal platelet-rich plasma, showing attachment of fibrin threads to clumps of activated platelets (× 22,000). (From Saleem A, Blifeld C, Saleh SA, et al.: Viscoelastic measurement of clot formation: A new test of platelet function. Ann Clin Lab Sci 13:115–124, 1983.)

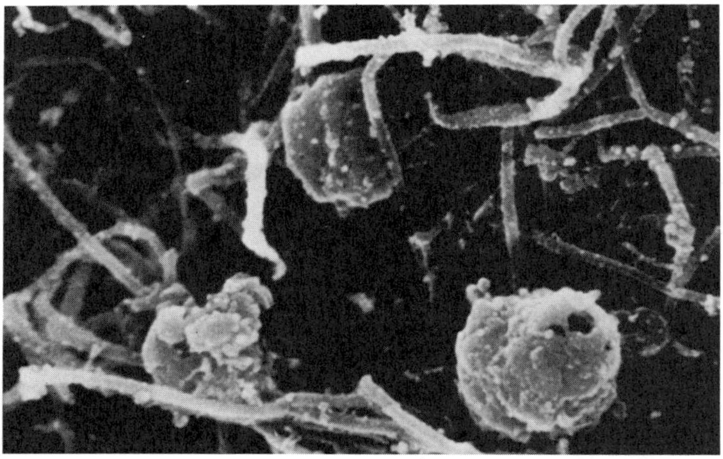

Figure 12–5. Scanning electron micrograph of recalcified platelet-rich plasma from a patient with platelet dysfunction, showing poor attachment of fibrin threads to inactive platelets (× 22,000). (From Saleem A, Blifeld C, Saleh SA, et al.: Viscoelastic measurement of clot formation: A new test of platelet function. Ann Clin Lab Sci 13:115–124, 1983.)

for TGT and signatures was each 5 per cent. He found that, for detection of hypercoagulable states, the combination of the two tests was more sensitive than PT, PTT, AT-III, or platelet counts. He measured the slope of primary wave and peak times of recalcified PPP and compared the results of the situation. From this, he concluded that the TGT and plasma clot impedance signature tests are practical, rapid, and useful for the detection and monitoring of the hypercoagulable state.

Microheparin Assay

Abbasi and Johnson developed a microheparin assay by adding 50 lambda of plasma and excess thrombin to a buffer solution containing the necessary clotting factors.[11] The presence of heparin slows down the rate of fibrin formation and affects the measured impedance of clot formation. Signatures were calibrated with known heparin concentration standards (Fig. 12–6).

They then determined the concentration of heparin in sick preterm infants who were at risk of developing either hemorrhagic or thrombotic events due to insertion of catheters for parenteral administration of drugs

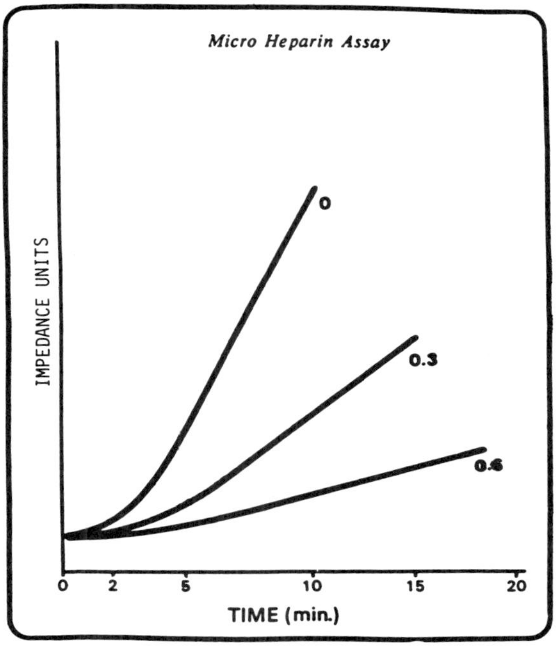

Figure 12–6. Sonoclot signature of heparinized infant plasma. The horizontal axis shows time, the vertical shows impedance unit. (From Abbasi S, Johnson L: A microheparin assay for sick preterm infants (abstract). Soc Pediatr Res 16:273A, 1982.)

and nutrition. These catheters usually contain heparin flush solution to prevent thrombosis. They pointed out that a circulating heparin level of 0.04 to 0.1 U/ml, which they considered the optimum range for minimizing the likelihood of clotting yet avoiding the risk of bleeding, is functionally equivalent to a PTT of approximately 40 to 60 sec. Only 3 of 20 sick preterm infants with indwelling catheters were found to be in the ideal range; 7 were too high and 10 were too low. They concluded that many infants are at a greater-than-necessary risk of both thrombosis and bleeding. They added that misinterpretation of the cause of bleeding (disseminated intravascular coagulation [DIC] vs. excessive heparin) may lead to inappropriate treatment that could result in increased risk of intraventricular hemorrhage.

Newlin et al. reported the use of this device for the control of heparin administration.[12] They pointed out that the quantification of heparin response in vitro is easily done by the recalcification of cellite-activated whole blood (ReACT) in this device. They constructed a two-point curve from samples containing 0 to 0.5 μ/ml of heparin prior to heparinization of the patient, and they compared the samples after heparin injection with the in vitro curve to determine the functional in vivo heparin concentration.

Other Uses

Blifeld et al. studied platelet function in neonates.[13] Blood was taken from the cord of normal and sick low birth weight neonates. In normal neonates, the blood had much shorter coagulation onset times and much steeper slopes than the adult normal values, whereas samples from the sick neonates all suggested diminished coagulation and platelet function. They concluded that the assessment of platelet function in the context of participation in ongoing coagulation may be more meaningful than results achieved using the conventional in vitro techniques.

The signature has been used in many other situations, such as the preoperative screening test of coagulation and the efficacy of treatment in Factor VIII deficiency; in progressive systemic sclerosis, atherosclerosis and hypercoagulability, thrombotic thrombocytopenic purpura, and procoagulant activity in cancer; in orthopedic surgery; in cases of altered blood viscosity as in polycythemia; and in dealing with dysfibrinogenemia.[14-17] The device produces a logarithmic response to viscosity (calibrated in centipoise) and has been used to measure viscosity of blood and plasma.[18]

THE SONOCLOT AND THE THROMBOELASTOGRAPH

The thromboelastograph (TEG) was introduced by Hartert in 1948 (see Ch. 11).[19] Both the Sonoclot and the TEG measure viscoelastic properties of the blood clot. While Sonoclot measures clot impedance to a vibrating probe, TEG measures the clot impedance by using a piston and rotating cuvette. Although the characteristic tracings produced by the two instruments appear different, there are similarities. Both measure recalcification time, rate of fibrin formation, clot strength, and clot lysis. Studies comparing the two instruments in comparable clinical situations have not been performed, and such a controlled study is needed. In the absence of such a study, we believe that the Sonoclot seems more sensitive to variations in platelet function.

References

1. Hattersley PG: Activated coagulation time of whole blood. JAMA 196:436–440, 1968.
2. Hayem G: Du sang et de ses alterations anatomiques. Paris: Masson, 1889, p. 323.
3. Wright AE: A note on certain improvements in the method of determining the condition of blood coagulability for clinical and experimental uses. Br Med J 1:237–241, 1894.
4. Lee RL, White PD: A clinical study of the coagulation time of blood. Am J Med Sci 145:493–496, 1913.
5. Koffman K: Der koaguloviskosimeter mit spezieller beruecksichtigung seiner klinischen verwendbarkeit fuer gerinnungsestimmungen des blutes. Z Klin Med 59:415–421, 1910.
6. Kugelmass IN: Contribution physico-clinique au mecanisme de la coagulation du san. Arch Int Physiol Biochim 21:139–146, 1923.
7. Von Kaulla KN, Ostendorf P, Von Kaulla E: The impedance machine: A new bedside coagulation recording device. J Med 6:73–87, 1975.
8. Saleem A, Blifeld C, Saleh SA, et al.: Viscoelastic measurement of clot formation: A new test of platelet function. Ann Clin Lab Sci 13:115–124, 1983.
9. Harker LA, Malpass TW, Branson HE, et al.: Mechanism of abnormal bleeding in patients undergoing cardiopulmonary bypass: Acquired transient platelet dysfunction associated with selective granule release. Blood 56:824–834, 1980.
10. Peck SD: Evaluation of the in vitro detection of the hypercoagulable state using the thrombin generation test and plasma clot impedance test. Thromb Haemost 42:764–777, 1979.
11. Abbasi S, Johnson L: A microheparin assay for sick preterm infants (abstract). The Society for Pediatric Research 16:273A, 1982.
12. Newlin F, Ens G, Leppke L, Hamstra R: Heparin control with the Sonoclot® (abstract). Am J Med Tech 44:508, 1978.
13. Blifeld C, Courtney JT, Gross JR: Assessment of neonatal platelet function using a viscoelastic technique. Ann Clin Lab Sci 16:373–376, 1986.
14. Gordon SG, Gilbert LC, Lewis BJ: Analysis of procoagulant activity of intact cells from tissue culture. Thromb Res 26:379–387, 1982.
15. Abbasi S, Johnson L: Microviscosity measurement using a mechanical impedance technique (abstract). The Society for Pediatric Research 16:197A, 1982.
16. Schreiber WE, Schmer G: Application of mechanical impedance measurements to the study of dysfibrinogens. J Lab Clin Med 104:494–500, 1984.
17. Schreiber WE, Schmer G: Fibrinogen Seattle II: Defective release of fibrinopeptide A in a slow clotting fibrinogen. Thromb Res 37:45–52, 1985.
18. Chandler WL, Schmer G: Evaluation of a new dynamic viscometer for measuring the viscosity of whole blood and plasma. Clin Chem 32:505–507, 1986.
19. Hartert H: Blutgerinnungsstudien mit der thrombelastographie, einem neuen untersuchungsverfahren. Klin Wochenchr 26:577–583, 1948.

CHAPTER 13

EFFECTIVE HEMOSTASIS IN THE CARDIAC SURGICAL PATIENT: Current Status

DAVID R. JOBES and NORIG ELLISON

Many of the problems introduced by applying cardiopulmonary bypass (CPB) to clinical management of heart disease have been successfully addressed. Homologous blood requirements have been drastically reduced, renal dysfunction has been all but eliminated, and excessive hemolysis is rarely seen. This monograph is, in part, a testimonial to the progress that has been achieved, exemplified by general agreement on practices throughout the chapters. These areas are (1) preoperative preparation (assessment and treatment) of non-CPB abnormalities of hemostasis, and (2) method of inducing, maintaining, and neutralizing heparin anticoagulation. This monograph is also a testimonial to the magnitude of one residual problem: *restoration of effective hemostasis following CPB*. Since the beginning of cardiac surgery with CPB in the 1950's, a puzzling phenomenon has plagued clinicians and researchers alike: Many patients do not resume normal hemostasis following neutralization of heparin anticoagulation. This phenomenon is so much a part of cardiac surgery that many have called this abnormal state "normal," thus focusing on those patients with sufficiently severe derangements to cause "clinically important" bleeding. This pragmatic categorization may be appealing to clinicians whose primary charge is to care for the patient at hand, but somewhat narrow for the intellectual challenge and wider applicability of understanding the basic problem. In addition, the current re-emphasis on transmission of viral illness via transfusion suggests that we can no longer accept this attitude. Clinically important bleeding must now include *any* need for transfusion.

There have been many attempts to define and solve the problem of effective hemostasis following CPB. An examination of the body of literature on this subject is often confusing, especially for the clinician. These frustrations are highlighted in this monograph by noting that virtually every contributing author begins by citing the multiplicity of identifiable contributing patient variables, limitations of investigative tools, and/or conflicting results of investigation and observation.

This chapter will summarize the general areas where a consensus exists and, in the areas of differing conclusions, will attempt to bring into focus our current understanding.

PREPARATION

The best method for detecting a hemorrhagic diathesis is a properly taken history; a most important part of the history is the hemostatic response to any prior surgical experience or medication. Any bleeding episode should be characterized by severity, site, duration, and presumed etiology, as well as similar episodes, age at onset of symptoms, and family history. Nearly all significant hereditary disorders of coagulation in an adult patient will be identified at this point. Knowing the existence of diseases coincidental to the reason for the proposed surgical procedure will further help to investigate acquired hemostatic problems. A singularly important area to identify during preparation is current drug therapy, especially anticoagulants and medication containing aspirin or other platelet-inhibiting drugs (see Ch. 6 and 7). The physical examination may support or add evidence of acquired disorders. Petechiae, ecchymosis, hemarthrosis, or prolonged active bleeding from puncture sites or wounds may be present.

The platelet count, prothrombin time (PT), activated partial thromboplastin time (aPTT), fibrinogen level, and bleeding time were suggested as a screening hemostatic profile for cardiac surgery in our 1981 review article. Many of our contributing authors in 1988 concur. Although no one test or pair of tests is sufficient to make a specific diagnosis or to rule out all potential causes of bleeding, a normal profile and negative history justify the assumption that a hemorrhagic diathesis is not present. The work of Salzman et al. (Ch. 9) suggests that incorporation of a Factor VIII:vWF assay into the profile is highly desirable. In their study, the preoperative level of Factor VIII:vWF correlated highly with postoperative blood loss.

The practice of ordering any routine battery of tests is certain to be questioned in this era of cost containment. At the University of Pennsylvania, in the last 6000 open-heart operations, one previously undiagnosed very mild Factor IX deficiency was first detected by a prolonged aPTT on a screening profile. Does this justify routine practice? Alone, it does not. However, the ability to discount a pre-existing hemorrhagic diathesis as a cause of excessive post-bypass bleeding is most reassuring in managing those patients who are bleeding excessively. With a negative history and a normal screening profile, that assumption is, indeed, valid. Furthermore, the values obtained with this profile will serve as baseline figures to which intraoperative values can be compared, e.g., a decrease in platelet count from 200,000 to 50,000 indicates a change in the wrong direction. Obviously, any abnormality discovered in the preparatory phase should result in definitive evaluation and correction. The vast majority of such problems are successfully dealt with in the elective patient population.

Unfortunately, the number of nonelective cardiac surgical patients for whom delays are impossible and who at the same time are at increased risk of hemostatic derangement is *increasing*! Antiplatelet therapy is more frequently used in patients with angina, who may require urgent surgery if they become unstable. Previous or ongoing heparin administration in patients who have unsuccessful percutaneous transluminal coronary artery angioplasty or who experience complications of that procedure may indicate the need for immediate surgery. Fibrinolytic therapy of acute coronary thrombosis to produce revascularization is becoming more common. However, immediate surgery will likely be performed if fibrinolytic therapy is unsuccessful. These situations dictate that we can only prepare and apply therapeutic intervention for use later in the course of surgery, usually after the adverse effects of CPB have been added. A high index of suspicion, a thorough understanding of new techniques (see Ch. 4), immediate meaningful laboratory assessment, and promptly available specific treatment must be applied for successful management.

INTENTIONAL INHIBITION OF HEMOSTASIS AND NEUTRALIZATION

Extracorporeal circulation systems are made of materials that stimulate the coagulation process to such an extent that inhibition is necessary to prevent pathological thrombus formation. Since the introduction of CPB, heparin has been used for this purpose. Heparin is a highly satisfactory drug because it is specific, and it has few side effects, virtually no time limit, and an available antidote. The only contraindication for heparin use in CPB, heparin-induced thrombocytopenia (HIT), has now been successfully managed (see Ch. 8). The most significant achievements in heparin use since the advent of CPB have been identification of variable patient response to dose, the effect of hypothermia in slowing heparin elimination, and the ability to monitor and maintain satisfactory anticoagulation with more precision (see Ch. 1 and 10). The impact of these achievements has meant an overall reduction in the total dose of heparin and, therefore, protamine, which has been associated with a reduction in postoperative blood loss and replacement. The reason may be the elimination of consumptive coagulopathy in some under-heparinized patients, and a reduction in the adverse effects of heparin-protamine complex on platelet function when excessive heparin has been used. It is generally accepted that initial and sequential measurements of heparin effect are desirable. The activated coagulation time (ACT) is the most widely used test for this purpose (see Ch. 1 and 10). Points of controversy in this area appear to be of minor clinical importance and involve the type of heparin chosen, the choice of test for monitoring heparin effect, and the place of monitoring circulating heparin concentration. The current use of heparin per se does not significantly contribute to problems in achieving hemostasis after bypass.

Prompt heparin neutralization after CPB is required for effective hemostasis, and protamine is almost exclusively utilized. Protamine is highly efficient in this regard but, unlike heparin, produces significant undesirable effects (see Ch. 2). Hypotension producing morbidity and even suspected mortality from ill-defined (allergic?) reactions has been documented. Fortunately, such reactions are uncommon. Since the neutralization of heparin by protamine depends on the amount of circulating drug (as opposed to heparin effect), an assessment of circulating heparin level is a more precise guide to protamine dose. Heparin rebound, which can occur following protamine neutralization, is easily detected and treated. This entity is seldom a documented reason for excessive postoperative bleeding. Further research in this area would lead to the formation of a more uniformly applied protamine dosage schedule than currently exists, or to the development of a better antidote.

Alternatives to heparin and protamine are few and of limited clinical value and experience. Absolute removal of a major element in the coagulation mechanism has been reported (defibrinogenation with ancrod). This technique has significant restrictions at this time and is limited in its application. The lack of development of suitable alternatives to heparin and protamine may reflect general acceptance and satisfaction with these drugs. However, the more widely recognized serious side effects of protamine, and the knowledge that heparin is not completely effective, may stimulate discovery of new and better techniques.

IDENTIFICATION OF HEMOSTATIC ABNORMALITIES AFTER NEUTRALIZATION OF HEPARIN

Much confusion and controversy exist at this point. A clear, uniform, clinical definition of "excessive" or "abnormal" bleeding to guide observations, to aid decision making, and to promote experimentation is lacking. The definition of excessive bleeding is quite arbitrary, and we recommend one approach. Table 13–1 is a thoroughly designed protocol that defines excessive bleeding as the need for reoperation. Patients who meet the levels indicated will have been in need of blood products for treatment. The effects of testing and the types of treatment could be assessed against such a table. The table could also provide a more reliable estimate of the incidence of problematic post-CPB bleeding.

Standard clinical laboratory assessments of the coagulation mechanism are virtually all abnormal with respect to the range of values obtained from healthy people. Highly refined laboratory research techniques have uncovered more abnormalities. The following potential causes of excessive bleeding are found to varying degrees in virtually all patients after CPB:

Fibrinolysis (proteolysis)
Decreased Factors V, VIII, XIII
Decreased fibrinogen
Decreased plasminogen
Decreased number of platelets (thrombocytopenia)
Decreased function of platelets
Complement activation

Much recent research has focused on the platelet. This complex vital component of the coagulation system has been carefully and exhaustively examined (see Ch. 6). In vitro analysis of platelet function under many different conditions has been performed. The result of this work is a long list of drugs and mechanical factors that are now known to alter platelet function. More than one or two of these drugs and/or conditions exist simultaneously in most of our patients with functional abnormalities, as confirmed by in vitro tests; it seems surprising that effective hemostasis is ever achieved. The authors would all seem to agree that platelets are structurally, functionally, and quantitatively abnormal as a result of CPB. There are varying degrees of abnormalities that result in excessive bleeding in some patients. We have no clinically useful assessment of platelets that is agreed upon to accurately predict the patient at risk, with the possible exception of extreme thrombocytopenia.

The only clearly agreed upon specific indication for platelet administration is thrombocytopenia *in a bleeding patient*. Another approach, namely inhibition/restoration of platelet function, has shown promise, and we may soon be able to see confirmatory results of widespread clinical trials with iloprost and desmopressin acetate (see Ch. 8 and 9). The obvious appeal is a decreased need for platelet transfusion with its attendant risks. In the meantime, clinicians have increasingly focused on platelet abnormalities and are more prone to use platelet transfusion on

TABLE 13–1. CHEST DRAINAGE CRITERIA FOR REOPERATION

Preoperative Weight (kg)	Hourly Amount (ml h^{-1}) No. of Successive Hours*			Total Amount (ml) Hour No.†	
	1	*2*	*3*	*4*	*5*
5.0	70	60	50	120	130
6.0	70	60	50	130	155
7.0	70	60	50	150	180
8.0	90	70	50	175	200
9.0	90	80	60	195	230
10.0	100	90	65	220	260
12.0	130	100	80	260	300
14.0	150	120	90	300	360
16.0	170	140	100	350	400
18.0	195	150	120	390	460
20.0	200	175	130	450	520
25.0	270	220	160	540	650
30.0	325	260	195	650	770
35.0	380	300	230	760	900
40.0	430	350	260	800	1,035
45.0	500	400	300	975	1,150
50.0	500	400	300	1,000	1,200

*Reoperation is advisable if the patient has bled the amount indicated in any 1 hour (column 1), the lesser amount in column 2 during each of any 2 successive hours, or the still smaller amount (column 3) in each of any 3 successive hours

†Reoperation is advisable if the patient has bled in total the amount indicated by the end of the fourth or fifth postoperative hour.

(From Kirklin JW, Barratt-Boyes BG: Cardiac Surgery. John Wiley & Sons, New York, 1986, p. 159. Reprinted by permission of John Wiley & Sons, Inc.)

an empirical basis in the bleeding post–CPB patient (see Ch. 5). The prophylactic administration of platelets has been decried by all. The role of platelet transfusion for suspected or measured platelet dysfunction must be viewed with some skepticism. Marengo-Rowe (see Ch. 3) restored hemostasis in a large series of bleeding patients after CPB without platelet administration, in spite of known platelet dysfunction in all patients, by using epsilon-aminocaproic acid (EACA) and cryoprecipitate (CP). This practice sharply contrasts with the introductory quotation from Harker in Chapter 6. Evidence that CP helps restore platelet function suggests that these points of view may not be so different. However, it is arguable that in regard to multiple donor exposure, the use of CP instead of platelets has little to offer.

Approximately 10 to 20 per cent of patients exhibit inadequate hemostasis of varying duration and severity, requiring multiple transfusions of blood products. Lack of benefit and increased risks associated with prophylactic administration of platelets and fresh frozen plasma (FFP) have led most, if not all, experts to caution against these and other forms of empirical or "shotgun" therapy. Specificity and rapid availability of results of a battery of evaluative tests that are serially repeated are stressed by every author. At the same time, all comment that this practice is difficult to achieve, although highly desirable, in the bleeding patient. This, we believe, represents the dilemma that confronts clinicians today. Faced with an unpredictably bleeding patient, the clinician must quickly choose a form of transfusion therapy. The delay in laboratory results and lack of specificity of those tests create the empirical management style that is prevalent, yet decried. We believe that a major challenge is to bring the laboratory more closely in line with the clinical setting with respect to both specificity of test and rapidity of results.

While research continues, we strive to clearly and quickly identify the patient at risk. The resurgence of interest in the thromboelastograph (TEG) suggests that it may be a useful qualitative screening device. It has proven valuable in detecting some specific abnormalities and in guiding therapy with more precision in hepatic transplantation. Modifications may make it as useful in cardiac surgical patients. As with the Sonoclot, the TEG produces a graphic representation of the dynamic clotting process and may be uniquely useful as a guide to therapy and decision making (see Ch. 11 and 12). An evaluation is currently underway to assess the impact of TEG-guided therapy on blood product utilization in cardiac surgical patients.

The future will produce at least partial solutions to the problem of altered hemostasis. Less reactive artificial surfaces combined with heparin and readily titratable platelet inhibitors will be the earliest mechanisms likely to reach the clinician. Desmopressin has a beneficial effect; its precise role awaits definition. At the present time, meticulous attention to preoperative hemostatic evaluations, ensuring an adequate response to pre–CPB heparin administration, intra–CPB maintenance of adequate heparin affect, and post–CPB protamine neutralization of heparin is the essential first step in securing effective hemostasis. The indication for platelets, FFP, or other specific therapeutic modalities will require more precise, timely evaluations of the coagulation system.

INDEX

Note: Page numbers in italics indicate a figure; page numbers followed by the letter t indicate a table.

Acquired immune dificiency syndrome (AIDS), transfusion-related, 72–73
Activated coagulation time (ACT), *2*, 3, 6–7, 76, 155–161
  history of, 155–156
  hypothermia and, 19–20, 157, 158, 159
    temperature correction for, *159*
  in heparin rebound, 160
  limitations of, 158–160, 160t, 174
  manual, 156
  operating room testing of, 3–4, 3t, *4*, *7*, 156–160
    automated, 3–4, *4*, *7*, 156–157
  preoperative, 114–115, 158
  protamine neutralization and, 158–160
  -TEG correlation, 169t, 175, 176t
  -WBCT relationship, 5–6
Activated partial thromboplastin time (aPTT), 5–7, 51–52, 51t, 52t
  after massive blood transfusion, 75–76, 75t
  CP and, 51
Acyl enzymes, as thrombolytic agents, 62
Adenosine diphosphate (ADP), platelet activation and, 89
Adenosine monophosphate, cyclic. See *Cyclic adenosine monophosphate (cAMP).*
Adenyl cyclase, 93–95, *94*
  stimulation of, 103–104
AIDS. See *Acquired immune deficiency syndrome (AIDS).*
Albumin, oxygenator platelet aggregation and, 97
Allergy, protamine, 21–24
    fish allergy and, 23
    prophylaxis against, 29–31, *30*
    vasectomy and, 23–24
  streptokinase, 61
Anaphylaxis, protamine, 16, 21–26
    avoidance of, 34–35, 34t
    prophylaxis of, 28–31, *30*
Ancrod, 32, 198
Angina pectoris, desmopressin and, 149
  von Willebrand's factor in, 148
Angioplasty, percutaneous transluminal coronary, emergency surgery in, 149
    desmopressin in, 149
Antibiotics, antiplatelet effects of, 102t, 114t
Anticoagulants. See also *Heparin; Protamine.*
  alternatives to, 31–32
  nonheparin, 32, 130
  oral, 129
Antiplasmin, 49, 57, 61, 63–64
Antithrombin-III (AT-III), 10
  deficiency of, 76
  protamine and, 17–18
aPTT. See *Activated partial thromboplastin time (aPTT).*
Arachidonic acid, platelet function and, 89, *90*
Aspirin, antiplatelet effects of, 102–103, 114t
    TEG monitoring of, 177
  bleeding time and, 116
  desmopressin with, 149
  in thrombocytopenia, 127, 130
AT-III. See *Antithrombin-III (AT-III).*

Biclot Elvi 816, 164
Bleeding. See also *Hemorrhage.*
  assessment of, 51–52, 51t, 52t, 75–76, 75t, *78*, 118
    investigative approach to, 46–47, *78*
    postoperative, 116–117, 198–201, 200t
    preoperative, 112, 114–116, 196–197
    Sonoclot, 187–189, 188–189t
    TEG, 174–177, 176t
  defined, 43
  excessive, 43, 118, 199, 200t
  fibrinolysis and, 48–51
  laboratory tests of, 44–45, 51–52, 51t, 52t, 73–76, 75t

Bleeding *(Continued)*
  management of, 50–53, 51t, 66, 74–76, 75t, 80
    desmopressin in. See *Desmopressin acetate.*
    FFP in, 74–76, 75t
    platelet transfusion in, 117–119
    "shotgun," 80–81
    surgical, 200t
  oxygenator type and, 43
  pathogenesis of, 44–47, 137–138
  patient characteristics and, 41–42, 112, 114–116, 196–197
  platelets and, 47–48, 112, 188–189, *190*, 199–200
  reoperation for, 200t
  thrombolytic therapy and, 61–62, 66
  type of surgery and, 42
  von Willebrand's factor and, 141, 147, *148*
Bleeding time, 115–116
  desmopressin and, 139
  in heparin-induced thrombocytopenia, *133*
Blood loss. See *Bleeding.*
Blood products, 69–83. See also specific product, e.g. *Cryoprecipitate (CP); Fresh frozen plasma (FFP).*
  complications with, 71–73, 79
  inappropriate use of, 76–77
  indications for, 73–76, 73t
  massive transfusion of, 74–75
    TEG in, 169
  platelet, 117–118
  "shotgun" therapy with, 80, 179, 200
  spontaneous heparin termination and, 32–33
  usage of, 69–70
    TEG guidance for, 171, 173, 179
  whole blood, 69
Blood transfusions. See also *Blood products.*
  massive, 74–75
    TEG in, 169
Bubble oxygenators. See *Oxygenators.*

Calcium, platelet function and, 89, 95
Calcium channel blocking agents, platelet effects of, 104
Calmodulin, 95
CAMP. See *Cyclic adenosine monophosphate (cAMP).*
Cancer, protamine in, 17
Cardiopulmonary bypass surgery, ACT in, 157–158
  bleeding after, *78*, 195–201. See also *Bleeding.*
  CP in, 80
Cardiopulmonary bypass surgery *(Continued)*
  desmopressin after, 145–149, *148*
  evaluation before, 112, 114–116, 196–197
  FFP in, 76–77
  fibrinolysis in, 48–50
  heparin in. See *Heparin.*
  platelet function during, 96–97, *98*, 99–101, 105–106, 111–112, 113t, 114–117, 199–200
    inhibition of, 101–105
      TEG monitoring of, 177
  platelet transfusion in, 117–119
  Sonoclot in, 187–189, 188–189t
  TEG in, 173–179, *176*, 176t
  thrombolytic therapy and, 66
  volume expansion and, 70, 77
Cardiotomy suckers, blood loss and, 52
  platelet dysfunction and, 100–101
Catastrophic pulmonary vasoconstriction, protamine and, 24–26, *25*
Cell membrane, platelet, 86–87, *87*
  drug effects on, 104–105
Chest drainage reoperation criteria, 200t
Children. See also *Infants.*
  heparin dose in, 5
Christmas disease, surgery in, 73–74
Clot formation time, Sonoclot, 185–187, *185*, 186t, *187*
  thromboelastographic, 166
Clot lysis times, 64–65
  thromboelastographic, 166
Clot strength, maximum, thromboelastographic, 166
Coagulation, disseminated intravascular, avoidance of, 4, 158
    fibrinolysis and, 48
    TEG diagnosis of, 173
Coagulation cascade, *6*, 88–89, 88t, 90, *91*
  measurement of, 168, 174, 176
Coagulation factors, 5, *6*. See also specific factors.
  assays of, 45
  bleeding variations and, 46
  deficiencies of, 73–74
    single donor plasma in, 77–78
    TEG data in, 168t
  postsurgical levels of, 77
Coagulation measurement, desirable characteristics for, 3t, 184t. See also specific measurement techniques.
Coagulation time, thromboelastographic, 164, 166
Coaguloviscosimeter, 183
Complement, in heparin-induced thrombocytopenia, 126–127
  protamine reaction and, 26
Coronary artery bypass grafting, desmopressin in, 149–150
  thrombolytic therapy and, 66

Corticosteroids, in thrombolytic therapy, 61
Cryoprecipitate (CP), 78–80
  after cardiopulmonary bypass, 80
  as glue, 79
  complications with, 79
  history of, 78–79
  in postsurgical bleeding, 50–52, 51t, 66, 80, 200
  indications for, 79
Cyclic adenosine monophosphate (cAMP), pharmacologic evaluation of, 103–104
  platelet activation and, 93–95, *94*, 127
Cyclo-oxygenase inhibition, 101–103, 102t, 130

DDAVP. See *Desmopressin acetate (DDAVP)*.
Deep venous thrombosis, 172
  heparin resistance and, 10
  TEG monitoring of, 170–172, 179
Desmopressin acetate (DDAVP), 119, 137–153, 177–179
  after cardiopulmonary bypass, 145–149, *148*
  clinical pharmacology of, 138–140
  dosage of, 148
  future uses for, 149–150
  hemostasis and, 144–145
  in hemophilia and von Willebrand's disease, 142–143
  in spinal fusion surgery, 144
  in storage pool deficiency, 144
  in uremia, 144–145
  indications for, 149–150
  side effects of, 140
  TEG monitoring of, 178–179, *178*
  von Willebrand's factor and, 141
Diabetes, protamine sensitivity in, 21–22
Dipyridamole, antiplatelet effects of, 103
    TEG monitoring of, 177
  desmopressin with, 149
Disseminated intravascular coagulation, avoidance of, 4, 158
  fibrinolysis and, 48
  TEG diagnosis of, 173
Donor plasma, single, 77–78
Drug(s). See also specific drugs.
  administration of. See *Drug administration*.
  platelet function and, 86t, 102t, 114t
  thrombocytopenia and, 86t, 101–105, 102t
Drug administration, of desmopressin, 139
  of heparin, 11
  of protamine, arterial vs. venous, 26–28
  of streptokinase, hemorrhage and, 66
Duke bleeding time technique, 115

EACA. See *Epsilon-aminocaproic acid (EACA)*.
Edema, pulmonary, FFP and, 73
    protamine and, 24
Elderly, acute phase reactions in, 149
  hemorrhage in, during thrombolytic therapy, 61
Emergency surgery, 197
Endoperoxides, 93
  inhibition of, 94, 102
Epsilon-aminocaproic acid (EACA), 63–64
  therapy with, 49–53, 51t, 66, 80
    in vitro TEG test of, 173, *174*
Euglobulin clot lysis time, 48, 49, 65, 173

Factor assays, pitfalls of, 45
Factor deficiencies, FFP in, 73–74
  single donor plasma in, 77–78
  TEG data in, 168t
Factor IIa, protamine and, 17–18
Factor V, postsurgical levels of, 77
Factor VIII, desmopressin and, 138, 142–143
  in whole blood, 75
Factor Xa assay, 7
FFP. See *Fresh frozen plasma (FFP)*.
Fibrin, plasminogen and, 64
  selective agents against, 62–63
Fibrin plate assay, 65
Fibrinogen, 64
  after massive blood transfusion, 75t
  clotting rate variations of, 44–45
  fibrinolysis and, 48–49
  low postoperative, 159–160
  platelet aggregation and, 96
Fibrinolysis, 4, 41, 48–51
  as proteolysis, 49–50
  clinical measurement of, 64–65
  compensated, 48–49
  inhibitors of, 63–64
  laboratory test changes in, 65, 65t
  local, 64
  physiology of, 57–64, *58*
  TEG diagnosis of, 173, *176*
  therapeutic. See *Thrombolytic therapy*.
  treatment of, 50–53, 51t, 52t
    in vitro TEG test of, 173, *174*
Fibrinolytic enzyme system, 57–64, *58*
  fibrinolysis and, 64
Fibrinolytic therapy. See *Thrombolytic therapy*.
Fish allergy, protamine reaction with, 23
Fresh frozen plasma (FFP), 70–77
  as protamine alternative, 33
  complications with, 71–73
  description of, 70
  fulminant pulmonary edema and, 73
  history of, 70

Fresh frozen plasma (FFP) *(Continued)*
in antithrombin-III deficiency, 76
in heparin resistance, 9–10
in immunodeficiencies, 76
in postsurgical bleeding, 50–53, 51t, 66, 74–76, 75t
in tetralogy of Fallot surgery, 47–48
in thrombotic thrombocytopenic purpura, 76
inappropriate use of, 76–77, 179
indications for, 73–76, 73t
single donor plasma vs., 78
usage of, 69–70
viral infections and, 71–73
Fulminant hepatitis, 72

Glanzmann's thrombasthenia, 144
Glycosylation, variations in, 45

Halothane, antiplatelet effects of, 104
Heart-lung bypass. See *Cardiopulmonary bypass surgery.*
Heart valve surgery, blood loss in, 42
von Willebrand's factor and, 147–148
Hematocrit, 51
Hemochron heparin control, 3–4, *4*, 156–157
blood loss and, 42–43
temperature correction nomogram for, 157, *159*
Hemodilution, thrombocytopenia and, 74, 99–100, 111–112
TEG parameters and, 171, *171*
Hemolysis, CP and, 79
FFP and, 71
Hemophilia, 46
CP in, 79–80
desmopressin in, 138–139, 142–143
factor concentrates in, 72
surgery in, 73–74
TEG tracing in, 165
Hemorrhage. See also *Bleeding.*
arrest of, 50–51, 80–81
desmopressin in, 146–147
platelet dysfunction and, 85
prediction of, 175–176, 176t
sudden, 52
TEG parameters in, 171, *172*
thrombolytic therapy and, 61–62, 65–66
Hemostasis, 195–201. See also *Bleeding.*
concepts of, 46
desmopressin and, 141, 144–145
investigative approach to, 46–47, *78*
von Willebrand's factor in, 141
HemoTec ACT, 157
Heparin, 1–14, 197–198
action of, 5
administration of, 11
Heparin *(Continued)*
alternatives to, 31–32, 129–130, 198
dosage of, 1–5
dose-response curve, *2*, 3–4
in children, 5
in heparin-induced thrombocytopenia, 131, *131*
units vs. milligrams, 10–11
history of, 1
postoperative assessment of, 52, 158–160
protamine titration and, 7–8, 16, 198. See also *Protamine.*
rebound of, 11–13, 11t, *12*, 18–19
ACT and, 160
heparin type and, 19
resistance to, 9–10, *9*, 10t
Sonoclot assay for, 191–192, *191*
spontaneous termination of, 32–33
testing effects of, 5–8, *8*, 155–161
by TEG, 172, 177
thrombocytopenia induced by, 123–135
clinical presentation of, 124
diagnosis of, 125–126, *125*
incidence of, 124–125
management of, 128–131, *132*
mechanism of, 126–128
units vs. milligrams of, 10–11
variations in response to, 2–3, 8
Heparinase, 33
Heparinoids, 130
Hepatitis, subclinical, 72
transfusion-related, 71–72
Hepcon System IV, 157
Hexadimethrine, as protamine alternative, *33*, 34
Histamine, protamine and, 20, 27
Hypercoagulability, Sonoclot in, 189, 191
TEG in, 168t, 170–172, 179
Hypocoagulability, 170–171
Hypofibrinogenemia, 159–160
Hypotension, protamine, 20–21, 20t
injection method and, 26–28
prophylaxis against, 29–31, *30*
Hypothermia, ACT and, 19–20, 157–159
temperature correction for, *159*
thrombocytopenia and, 100
Hypovolemia, FFP for, 69–70, 77

Iloprost, *98*, 103–104, 127, *128*, *129*, 130–131
Immunodeficiency, acquired, transfusion-related, 72–73
secondary, FFP in, 76
Immunoglobulin G (IgG), platelet-associated, 126
Impedance measurement, Sonoclot, 184–185
Indomethacin, antiplatelet effects of, 101–103, 102t

Infants, heparin dose in, 5
heparin levels in, 191–192, *191*
platelet function in, 192
Insulin, protamine and, 16
Intravascular coagulation, disseminated, avoidance of, 4, 158
fibrinolysis and, 48
TEG diagnosis of, 173
Isoproterenol, 104
Ivy bleeding time technique, 115

Jaundice, 72

Laboratory tests. See also specific tests.
after massive blood transfusion, 74–76
baseline, 51–52
for bleeding assessment, 51–52, 51t, 52t, 75–76, 75t, 78, 118
postoperative, 116–117, 198–201
preoperative, 114–116, 196–197
for hypercoagulability, 189–190
pitfalls of, 44–45, 50
-TEG correlation, 166, 168, 169t, 175–176
thrombolytic therapy changes in, 65t
Leukocytes, protamine reactions and, 25–26
Liver transplantation, TEG coagulation changes during, *167*, 169–170

Membrane oxygenators. See *Oxygenators*.
Myocardial infarct, von Willebrand's factor and, 148–149

Neonates, heparin levels in, 191–192, *191*
platelet function in, 192
Non-A, non-B hepatitis, 72
Nonsteroidal antiinflammatory agents, antiplatelet effects of, 101–103, 102t

ORG 10172, 130
Organelle zone, 88–89, 88t
Oxygenators, air-blood interface in, 99
blood loss and, 43
in tetralogy of Fallot surgery, 47–48
platelet aggregation and, 96–97, *98*, 99–100, 103–104, 112

Partial thromboplastin time (PTT), 51–52, 51t
after massive blood transfusion, 75
fibrinolysis and, 65, 65t
-TEG correlation, 169t
Percutaneous transluminal coronary angioplasty, desmopressin in, 149
emergency surgery in, 197

Phosphodiesterase inhibition, 102t, 103–104
Phosphorylation, 94, *94*
Plasma, fresh frozen. See *Fresh frozen plasma (FFP)*.
platelet-rich vs. platelet-poor, Sonoclot of, 185–187, *185*, 186t, *187*
single donor, 77–78
Plasmin, 59
assays of, 59
bleeding and, 61
inhibitor of, 49, 57, 61, 63–64
streptokinase and, 60
Plasminogen, 49, 57–59, *59*, 64
activators of, 57, 60–63, 140
digestive products of, 58
fibrin and, 64
inhibitors of, 57, 60–61
lysine-binding sites in, 58, *59*
Platelet(s), 85–109
activation of, 89–91, *90–92*, 93–96, *94*
inhibition of, 101–105, 102t, 119, 130–131
heparin-induced, 126–128
aggregation of, 48, 91, *91*, 93
during cardiopulmonary bypass, 96–97, 112
heparin-induced. See *Thrombocytopenia, heparin-induced*.
inhibition of, 101–105, 102t, 127, *129*, *131*
measurement of, *92*, 116, 125–126, *125*
anatomy of, 86–89, *87*, 88t
cardiopulmonary bypass and, 96–97, *98*, 99–101, 105–106, 111–112, 113t, 114–119, 114t, 199–200
concentrated, as protamine alternative, 33
destruction of, 112
disease and, 114
drugs and, 86t, 102t, 114t
excessive bleeding and, 47–48, 112, 188–189, *190*, 199–200
Sonoclot analysis of, 185–187, *185*, 186t, *187*
TEG analysis of, 177
transfusions of, 117–118, 119, 199–200
autologous, 118
in tetralogy of Fallot surgery, 47–48
prophylactic, 118–119
Platelet count, 51–52, 51t, 113t, 115, 118. See also *Thrombocytopenia*.
after massive blood transfusion, 74
bleeding time and, 47–48, 115
in heparin-induced thrombocytopenia, *132*
protamine and, 24–25
Platelet factor 4 (PF_4), low affinity, 97
Platelet-associated IgG, 126
Plateletcrit, 116

Prophylaxis, before protamine administration, 28–31, *30*
  for fibrinolysis, 49
  with FFP, 69, 200
  with platelet transfusion, 118–119, 200
Prostacyclin, 97, 99, 103, 127, *128*
  desmopressin and, 145
Prostaglandins, *128*
  antiplatelet effects of, 103–104, 127
Prostanoids, 103, 130–131
Protamine, 15–39, 198
  ACT monitoring of, 158–160
  alternatives to, 31–35, 198
  anaphylactoid reaction to, 16, 21–26
  arterial vs. venous injection of, 26–28
  as anticoagulant, 17–18
  dosage of, *2*, 3–5, *4*, 19–20
    priming, 30
  heparin rebound and, 11–13, 11t, *12*, 18–19, 198
    heparin type and, 19
  history of, 15–16
  hypotension and, 20–21
    injection method and, 26–28
  idiosyncratic reactions to, 20–26, 20t
    avoidance of, 34t
  insulin and, 16, 21
  preparation of, 15
  pretreatment approach with, 28–31
    priming, 29–31, *30*
  pulmonary edema and, 24
  pulmonary vasoconstriction and, 24–26, *25*
  sensitization to, 21–24
    cross-reacting antigens in, 23–24
    in diabetes, 21–22
    prior exposure and, 22–23, 22t
    prophylaxis against, 28–31, *30*
  thrombocytopenia and, 17, 101
  titration of, 7–8, 16, 198
  toxicity of, 16, 20–26
    avoidance of, 34–35, 34t
Proteolysis, fibrinolysis as, 49–50
Prothrombin time (PT), 51–52, 51t, 52t, 77
  after massive blood transfusion, 74–75
  fibrinolysis and, 65, 65t
  preoperative, 114–115
  -TEG correlation, 169t
Prourokinase, 57, 62
PT. See *Prothrombin time (PT).*
PTT. See *Partial thromboplastin time (PTT).*
Pulmonary edema, FFP and, 73
  protamine and, 24
Pulmonary vasoconstriction, catastrophic, protamine and, 24–26, *25*

Reaction time, thromboelastographic, 164
Rh factor, platelet transfusions and, 117–118
Ristocetin, 138

Secretory granules, 88–89, 88t
  during cardiopulmonary bypass surgery, 100
Serotonin release, in heparin-induced thrombocytopenia, 126, 127, *129*
Snake venom, 32
Sol-gel zone, 87–88, *87*
Sonoclot, 76, 183–193, 201
  after cardiopulmonary bypass, 187–189, 188–189t, 201
  equipment for, *184*
  heparin assay by, 191–192, *191*
  history of, 183
  in hypercoagulable states, 189, 191
  in neonates, 191–192, *191*
  interpretation of, 185–187, *185*, 186t, *187*
  technique for, 184–185
  thromboelastography and, 192–193
Spinal fusion surgery, desmopressin in, 144
Storage pool deficiency, desmopressin in, 144
Streptokinase, 57, 60
  allergic reaction to, 61
  hemorrhage and, 66
  hypofibrinogenemia and, 159–160
    TEG measurement of, *165*
  plasminogen activation by, 60, *61*
"Stress" hormones, coagulation changes and, 170–171
Surgeon, blood loss variations and, 42–43
Surgery. See also specific procedure.
  after thrombolytic therapy, 65–66
  coagulation changes during, *167*, 169–173
  desmopressin in, 142–143, 149–150
  emergency, 197
  evaluation before, 112, 114–116, 196–197
  in uremia, 143–144
  proteolysis after, 49–50
  TEG in, 169–173
  thrombocytopenia and, 86t, 113t
    heparin-induced, 129–131, *131–133*, *132*
  variations in blood loss during, 42–43

Tachyphylaxis, desmopressin, 140
TEG. See *Thromboelastography (TEG).*
Tetralogy of Fallot surgery, 47–48
Thrombin, protamine and, 17–18
Thrombin generation test (TGT), 189, 191
Thrombin time (TT), 51–52, 51t
  after massive blood transfusion, 74–75
  fibrinogen variations and, 44
  fibrinolysis and, 65, 65t

Thrombocytopenia, desmopressin in, 145
  dilutional, 74, 99–100, 111–112, 171
  drugs causing, 102t, 105, 112
  heparin-induced, 123–135
    clinical presentation of, 124
    diagnosis of, 125–126, *125*
    incidence of, 124–125
    management of, 128–131, *131–133*, 132
    mechanism of, 126–128
  hypothermia and, 100
  platelet transfusion and, 118–119, 199
  protamine, 17, 101
  surgery and, 86t, 99–100, 113t
  TEG data in, *165*, 168t
Thromboelastograph coagulation analyzer, 164
Thromboelastography (TEG), 76, 163–181, 201
  algorithm for interpretation of, 168t
  blood product usage and, 171, 173, 179
  characteristic tracings by, *165*
  correlation of data from, 166, 168, 169t, 175–176
  equipment for, 163–164, *164*
  fibrinolysis diagnosis by, 173, *174*, *176*
  future applications of, 179
  in cardiopulmonary bypass surgery, 173–179, *176*, 176t, 201
  in liver transplantation, *167*, 169–170
  methodology of, 163–164, 166, 168t
  perioperative, 169–173, *174*
  postoperative, 177
  Sonoclot and, 192–193
Thrombogenesis, 3
Thrombolytic therapy, 57–68
  contraindications to, 61–62
  fibrin-selective agents in, 62–63
  fibrinolysis measurement in, 64–65
    TEG and, *165*
  hemorrhage and, 61–62, 65–66
  laboratory test changes in, 65t
  new agents in, 62–63
  streptokinase in, 60, *61*
  TEG monitoring of, 173
  surgery after, 65–66
  urokinase in, 60
Thrombosis, deep venous, 172
  heparin resistance and, 10
  TEG monitoring of, 170–172, 179
Thrombotic thrombocytopenic purpura, FFP in, 76
Thromboxane A_2, in heparin-induced thrombocytopenia, 127
  inhibition of, 102–103
  platelet activation and, 93
  synthesis of, 89, *90*
Tissue-type plasminogen activator (t-PA), 57, 62–63
  desmopressin and, 139–140
Tissue-type plasminogen activator (t-PA) *(Continued)*
  inhibitors of, 63
Titration, heparin, 3–4
  protamine, 7–8, 16, 198
Toluidine blue, as protamine alternative, 33–34
t-PA. See *Tissue-type plasminogen activator (t-PA).*
Transfusions, blood. See also *Blood products.*
  massive, 74–75
    TEG in, 169
  platelet. See *Platelet(s), transfusions of.*
Transplantation, liver, TEG coagulation changes in, *167*, 169–170
Tri-F titer, 51–52, 51t
TT. See *Thrombin time (TT).*

Uremia, desmopressin in, 144–145
Urokinase, 57–60
  inhibitors of, 63
  thrombolytic therapy with, 60

Valvular heart disease surgery, blood loss and, 42
  von Willebrand's factor and, 147–148
Vasectomy, protamine reaction after, 23
  prophylaxis against, 28
Vasoconstriction, pulmonary, protamine and, 24–26, *25*
Vasodilation, desmopressin and, 140
Viral infections, CP and, 79
  FFP and, 71–73
Viscoelastic measurement. See *Sonoclot.*
Vitamin K, warfarin effect and, 7
Volume infusion, FFP for, 69–70, *77*
  protamine injection method and, 27
von Willebrand's disease, 79
  desmopressin in, 138–139, 142–143
    contraindication to, 143
    TEG monitoring of, 178–179, *178*
von Willebrand's factor, 138, 141
  assays for, 147
  desmopressin and, 141
  in hemostasis, 141, 147, *148*

Warfarin, effect of, reversal of, 74
WBCT. See *Whole blood coagulation time (WBCT).*
Whole blood, 69
  massive transfusions of, 74–75
Whole blood clot lysis time, 64
Whole blood coagulation time (WBCT), 5–7
  -ACT relationship, 5–6
  protamine and, 17